PRAISE FOR

Throw Away the Scale

"Reading this book feels like finally having an unhurried, compassionate conversation with your medical provider. With wisdom from years of treating chronic illness, Magdalena invites us to stop chasing a number on the scale and start building a strong body and joyful life. This book makes you want to put it down and start exercising."

—**CYNTHIA GRIFFITH**, MPAS, PA-C, editor of *Journal of Dermatology for Physician Assistants*

"*Throw Away the Scale* is a refreshing guide to true health and wellness—one that prioritizes how we feel over how much we weigh. It invites readers to tune into their bodies, eat mindfully, prioritize sleep, and move with joy. What resonated most with me is its empowering view of exercise—not as a tool for losing weight, but for feeling more energized, clearheaded, and emotionally balanced. As a health coach, I've seen how these simple habits help my clients feel better, regain their energy, and enjoy life more. This book is a must-read for anyone seeking a more intuitive and sustainable path to health."

—**ANGÉLIQUE LAVOIE**, health coach

"In *Throw Away the Scale*, Magdalena Chavez offers more than a medical perspective—she offers a path toward healing that honors the dignity of the human person. This book is grounded in compassion and insight as it calls us to see health not through the lens of numbers, but through the lens of wholeness. As a pastor, I see how often people carry silent burdens of shame about their bodies. This book is a liberating message that echoes a deeper truth of our faith: that we are fearfully and wonderfully made (Psalm 139:14), and that true vitality begins with the care of the whole person—body, mind, and spirit. I warmly recommend this book to anyone seeking not only better health, but a more grace-filled life."

—REVEREND FATHER JACOB DANKASA, PhD, author of *Faith, Not Convenience: 17 Reflections for Spiritual Consistency* and pastor at Holy Family of Nazareth Catholic Church

"Magdalena Chavez manages to blend cutting-edge science, common sense, and plenty of inspiration into one fantastic read that flips the traditional model of health on its head. She makes the case that motion isn't optional, it's essential, and that the scale isn't telling you everything you need to know about your health. If you're interested in improving and maintaining your health until your very last breath (at a very advanced age), read this book."

—DAVID STARBUCK SMITH, author of *Align, Feel, Heal: An Integrated Solution to Eliminating Chronic Pain*

THROW AWAY THE SCALE

Throw Away the Scale: Measuring Life in Vitality Instead of Pounds

by Magdalena Chavez, PA-C

© Copyright 2025 Magdalena Chavez, PA-C

ISBN 979-8-88824-846-1

All rights reserved. No part of this publication may be reproduced, stored in a retrieval system, or transmitted in any form or by any means—electronic, mechanical, photocopy, recording, or any other—except for brief quotations in printed reviews, without the prior written permission of the author.

Cover and book design by Lauren Sheldon

Published by

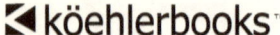

3705 Shore Drive
Virginia Beach, VA 23455
800-435-4811
www.koehlerbooks.com

THROW AWAY the SCALE

Measuring Life in Vitality
Instead of Pounds

MAGDALENA CHAVEZ, PA-C

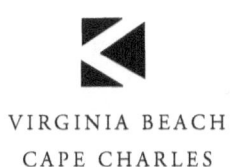

VIRGINIA BEACH
CAPE CHARLES

TABLE OF CONTENTS

Introduction..ix

CHAPTER 1
A Long Time Coming (The Backstory).......................1

CHAPTER 2
Getting Back to Nature.. 6

CHAPTER 3
Neurochemicals 16

CHAPTER 4
Hormones 33

CHAPTER 5
Digestion 39

CHAPTER 6
Memory... 46

CHAPTER 7
What About Pain?... 52

CHAPTER 8
Getting Going 67

CHAPTER 9
Food: Both Fuel and Pleasure 74

Conclusion... 85
Acknowledgments... 89
Bibliography 91

INTRODUCTION

Our obsession with weight is actually making us less healthy, and often, even fatter. True, some rare individuals among us are able to place a focus on their weight or BMI (body mass index) and maintain healthy levels through simple changes in their diet and exercise routine. But for the majority of us, the scale is a defeating metric that, more often than not, leads to frustration, anger, the backlash of weight gain, and even more frustration.

We need to make an important distinction between "weight" and "health." They are not the same! In my work as an internal medicine PA, I have several patients who are objectively "skinny" but get winded climbing a flight of stairs or taking their kids to the park. On the other hand, I have patients who are unhappy with their weight and may fall on the overweight or even obese side of a BMI chart but are more fit than their categorically skinny counterparts. True, our so-often-mentioned BMI (a ratio of one's weight to height) is a marker of our overall health, but weight is only *one* marker among many. And yet, it somehow receives an outsized focus in terms of health measures.

Medical providers may contribute to this imbalance even further. We discuss several factors that affect our patients' health, including blood pressure, blood glucose (sugar), cholesterol levels, sleep, and mood, which are all important in maintaining a healthy body, mind, and heart, and yet we seem to spend much less time concentrating on these factors compared to the amount of time we spend discussing weight. Why is that? Perhaps it's become ingrained in our modern medical practice that weight is the single most important factor in our overall health, but weight alone is not an accurate measure of health, and other aspects, particularly our *mental* health, have suffered as a result.

To illustrate the difference between health and weight, think of a friend or acquaintance you may know that fits this common picture: They have a healthy BMI on paper, but often complain about feeling sluggish, bloated, or run-down, and they have frequent aches and pains. Worse yet, when we monitor the lab work of individuals such as these, we often find elevated inflammatory factors, elevated blood sugar, and abnormal cholesterol. People sometimes refer to this as "skinny fat." They may also suffer from mood disorders such as depression, anxiety, or insomnia.

You probably likewise know many people, like I do, that carry a few extra pounds but seem healthier, and dare I say happier, because they maintain healthy habits in terms of their diet, exercise, and sleep. They have more energy. Their labs look healthier. Often, people in this category are at least close to a medically ideal weight, but not always, and it is not their main focus.

Then there's the majority of us—who focus on the scale. We struggle with weight as the main measure of our health, then feel defeated when we do not see progress as soon as we would like. So we give up altogether and sink into unhealthy diet habits and a sedentary lifestyle, ending up not only overweight but also fatigued, achy all over, and at higher risk for health complications like elevated blood pressure, high blood sugar, heart disease, and even some cancers.

In my clinical practice, I see a lot of patients who are concerned about their weight. Unfortunately, in so many of these office visits, I hear patients talk about the truly *un*healthy things they have tried in order to achieve their "ideal weight." These include crash diets that deprive the body of needed nutrients or taking medications that cause harm in the form of insomnia, stomach pain, palpitations, and elevated blood pressure—all in the name of dropping those few pounds. I've even heard patients say that they are intentionally stopping exercise because they *want* to lose some muscle mass in order to lower the number on the scale.

What's even sadder is that I totally understand their drive to do this, and I do think that we as medical providers may be contributing to this mindset. I would hope that clinicians are taking a balanced approach when discussing lifestyle factors that affect a patient's health, but too often these conversations are cut short, and we instead resort to the fast and easy phrases like "you need to drop ten/twenty/fifty pounds."

Few of our patients are successful in achieving that weight loss, and for those that are not, the guilt and failure sometimes keep them from coming back to the clinic altogether. Some of our patients who are successful in losing the weight are surprised to see that they still feel fatigued or depressed. There is a tendency to think that "skinny" means "in shape." Patients have often told me that they get out of breath walking through the parking lot or taking their kids on a field trip, then state that if they could just get bariatric surgery or medicine to lose the weight, they would have energy. Some patients even suggest that losing weight would cure their depression. But these claims are far from true! While someone may get a temporary boost of self-confidence, weight loss alone will not solve a mood disorder, nor will it automatically give you energy. *How* someone loses weight, on the other hand, may indeed help with these goals.

I have also met patients who tell me they plan to lose weight by going on a particular diet they heard about and are dreading, or that they bought a gym membership even though they hate going to the gym. I can't help but wonder: Why would you force yourself to do something you don't enjoy? And more importantly, if you don't enjoy it, do you think you will be able to stick with it in the long term?

It's disheartening when patients feel they have to force themselves to do something unpleasant in order to be healthy. It shouldn't be this way—taking care of your health may require some effort, but ultimately, it should *feel good*.

The fact is that weight is just one factor of many, and true health is a combination of many factors, including cardiovascular endurance, systemic inflammation, hormone balance, and psychological health.

CHAPTER 1

A Long Time Coming (The Backstory)

I have to admit right off the bat that I have fallen into the pitfall of weight obsession for most of my life, and it has taken years of trial and error, clinical training, and continuous practice to reverse that singular focus on counting calories and pounds.

My childhood started out like most. My mother's Midwestern-style of cooking meant that we ate mostly home-cooked meals, but with a heavy emphasis on meat and potatoes, and if there was "salad" served, it might have been made of Jell-O and/or a mixture of fruit covered in whipped cream. Of course, back then, I didn't have any concept of what healthy or unhealthy meant, aside from thinking that healthy meant you were not home sick with the flu. I was an active kid though, running around with my neighborhood friends almost daily and walking to and from the community pool as often as I could in the summertime.

I did notice, even at a young age, that my mother seemed very preoccupied by her own weight. She would sometimes make a pact with friends to start a fitness routine or get the latest home aerobics video in the name of losing weight. I am sure that she, like any mother, never intended to pass on her own insecurities to me, but I couldn't help but look at my own thighs while she measured, poked, and prodded at her own.

As I mentioned, I loved being active, as many kids do. I joined the swim team as early as I could remember and took gymnastics for a few years after expressing interest in dance, at which my parents told me that my body type was more suited for gym than for ballet. (Again, they had no intention of body-shaming, but the message of shame clearly landed, and I would even say lingered.) I enjoyed the activity for the sake of it and for the sense of accomplishment that came with sports. I eventually rose to a highly competitive level in swimming, which meant practicing several hours a day, sometimes twice a day before and after school. And here again came a focus on weight that occupied more than a healthy amount of attention. One of my swim team coaches introduced weigh-ins between swim workouts and "dry-land" or weight-lifting workouts at least once a week. After standing on the scale in front of him and the entire coed swim team, I was mortified to learn that I weighed thirty pounds more than I remembered weighing previously (and what I thought I *should* weigh at the time.) Never mind the fact that we had been adding thirty to sixty minutes of weight training several days a week on top of swimming laps and doing drills for ninety minutes to two hours a day—or that I now had shoulder muscles to rival any cartoon villain. I went home and cried that evening, resolved to get the weight back off even if that meant crash dieting. Of course this was a terrible idea, which not only did *not* lead to lasting weight loss, but did leave me feeling so exhausted that I could barely survive a swim practice and found myself falling asleep in classes.

I also started getting injured at an unusual rate, which at the time I took as a sign of weakness and further proof that I needed to work harder. So I ate even less. In hindsight, I now know that this was my body crying for help (and proper nutrition)! Between the injuries and my ever-increasing fatigue, my swimming career came to an end, probably much sooner than it needed to.

Somewhere in the aftermath of walking away from swimming and in the midst of college life, I began to rediscover exercise and also that eating healthy foods actually made my body feel better. True, I also reached my peak weight at this time, as I gained not only the normal "freshman fifteen" or "sophomore twenty" but the dreaded "ex-athlete thirty." I wasn't proud of my weight, but at the same time, I actually did feel better in my own body. I had more energy and more joy in my day than I had felt in years.

This trend continued through most of my young adult life. I remained slightly overweight for my barely-over-five-foot height, but I stayed fairly active, taking up dance classes at a local community college, enjoying on-again-off-again relationships with gyms, taking walks to spend some time with my little brother, and then going on short jogs to get my dog some much-needed exercise. I eventually got back into swimming and tried my hand at a triathlon in my late twenties, which was an exhilarating experience that I still hope to repeat someday. I'm not fast on a bike or on the run, but I found that it didn't matter. Many of the people there were at various levels of fitness and speed, and they all seemed so positive and encouraging. The atmosphere was simply amazing, just so full of energy. And the runner's high was literally intoxicating!

I found that during PA school I had much less time for exercise, and definitely not enough time to train for a triathlon, but I made it a priority to stick with some amount of cardiovascular exercise throughout my graduate education and becoming a parent to young children. Finding the time at all was not easy, but I definitely felt better for it. I would also say that, especially in graduate school, I noticed that I needed some mental breaks, and physical activity felt even more essential during this time. Plus, the more I learned about the human body and brain, I understood more and more why I felt better and actually had more energy when I exercised.

But still, I struggled with getting my weight down to what I thought to be a healthy number. Sometimes I would blame my muscular frame, or my German heritage, but the scale never seemed to get within ten to fifteen pounds of where BMI charts said I should be, even during triathlon training. And at times, I'm sad to say, I would let my frustration with my weight get the better of me, and I would want to give up altogether.

If this sounds familiar, then I'm happy to let you know that you are not alone.

Ironically, it was early in the COVID pandemic lockdown of 2020 that I found my healthiest self, and a new relationship with exercise. I, like many people stuck at home and nervous about what was going on in the world, needed some major stress relief. Around this time, a friend of mine that lived in the same neighborhood messaged me that she was feeling stressed and anxious as well. She had been a runner, and although running had never been my favorite form of exercise, when she suggested that we go for a socially distanced run outside to blow off some steam, I gladly accepted.

This became our new routine through most of the spring and summer of 2020. I spent all day trying to work at home, which meant struggling with technology through telemedicine visits and simultaneously supervising my young kids' Zoom classes and schoolwork, all while trying to maintain some sense of calm with an ever-growing amount of uncertainty in the world and ever-more rambunctious, cooped-up children. I began to relish my standing date to unplug and get outside for a run at four o'clock every afternoon. I would joke with my spouse and friends that those runs kept me sane, but there is probably more truth to that statement than I realized at the time.

As the schools and clinics began to reopen along with the rest of the world, I had to shift my running to the wee hours of the morning before work rather than after it, but by then I was hooked. I knew that running would somehow leave me feeling both calm and exhilarated, and I was definitely not going to give it up.

Of course, along the way, I had also developed some of the strongest legs I had ever had in my life, and I did lose a couple of pounds over the course of that year. I also developed a series of goals, chasing after a new distance or certain speed, and it felt amazing to meet those milestones. More than anything, the driving force getting me out of bed at five o'clock in the morning was the idea that my mood would be improved for the rest of the day. I also noticed that I slept better on the days that I ran, and that I actually had more energy for the day after a thirty-minute run versus hitting the snooze button for an extra thirty minutes of shut-eye.

A few years older now, I still notice the scale going up and down a bit, and sometimes, even with a consistent exercise routine, my clothes will feel tight after too much holiday eating, but whatever weight fluctuation may come, my exercise routine is now one of the most essential parts of my day. One day, feeling good about my body, I stepped on the scale to check my "progress" only to realize, in fact, that I had not lost a single pound. Yes, I briefly fell into the trap. I felt so defeated that day. But by the next day, it didn't matter. I still felt that if I got up and out of bed, my day would just be better. I would be able to focus more effectively at work; I would be calmer with my kids when I got home; I would move more easily in my body throughout the day; and I would rest more soundly that night.

My body has discovered that this amazing medicine called exercise is the one thing that helps me feel happier, stay focused more easily, sleep more deeply, and actually feel fewer aches and pains. That alone makes for a miracle treatment that we should all be lining up to take! But add these perks to all the medical benefits that we know *should* motivate us to exercise (like lowering blood sugar and preventing cardiovascular disease), as well as the fact that, yes, at the end of the day, exercise also improves physical appearance, and it is no wonder that bodies in motion tend to stay in motion.

CHAPTER 2

Getting Back to Nature

Our bodies are literally made for movement. Kids exercise all the time, but they don't think of it as a chore the way most adults do, and they don't call it exercise. They call it play. We grow up naturally inclined to move our bodies, to run around and play tag or ride bikes or jump into swimming pools. Anyone who has spent a significant amount of time around young children has probably noticed how much they automatically move their bodies, constantly looking for activities or games to play. On the other hand, anyone who has spent time with a young child who has been cramped up inside for one reason or another (bad weather, for example) has probably also noticed that they tend to get quite cranky. It does not feel good to sit still for long periods of time, and our bodies naturally know that from the time we are young.

Likewise, anyone who has spent time around young kids has probably noticed that they sleep deeply. Some of this likely has to do with their growth and development, as it requires a tremendous amount of energy to grow, but much of their ability to sleep deeply also comes from their high activity level during the day. Children who are not given the opportunity to move and play throughout the day tend to have a more difficult time getting to sleep and staying asleep. Again, they just know that they need to move regularly in order for their bodies and minds to function comfortably.

As we age, we begin to occupy our time with other concerns and activities, and exercise (or movement in general) becomes less of a priority. We tend to become sedentary until exercise turns into something difficult that we *have to* get through, rather than something fun. We have lost the natural sense of joy that comes with movement.

The trend toward inactivity seems to be starting at an earlier and earlier age, as I am now seeing adolescent and teenage patients who have already given over to a sedentary lifestyle. Although factors such as bad weather and decreased time for physical movement in the school day plays a role, there is no doubt that we are seeing our younger and younger patients trade in physical play for sedentary activities such as video games or scrolling through social media, and it has been having a detrimental effect on both the physical and mental health of our youth. The trade-off of physical activity for increasingly sedentary play shows up now in our children's mood and behavior as well as medical conditions. I have encountered type 2 diabetes and high blood pressure at an alarming rate among my young patients, and I am also seeing a shocking number of these patients complain of anxiety, depression, and insomnia. No doubt that both of these trends are disturbing, and can be linked, at least in part, to decreased physical movement.

When we look at the rest of the natural world, we also see constant movement. It is not only children that show us the natural inclination to move and play, but the animal world demonstrates this as well. If you have a pet at home, then you've seen their need to move and play, whether it be through a game of fetch or taking a walk, or a cat climbing their tower. Wild animals display this as well. Dolphins jump in and out of the water for play; primates run, swing, and climb; and birds fly, dive, and swoop for fun as well as in search of food. An animal who is sedentary for any length of time (outside of hibernation) is presumed to be sick! Why would we accept this behavior in humans?

We as human beings, at any age, are also animals who are made to move, and we used to do just that as part of our basic survival.

For most of human history, we moved our bodies as we hunted, gathered, or farmed food. We labored to build and maintain our shelter, and to create many of the things we needed or wanted. We walked to see our friends and family. We entertained ourselves with games and pastimes that involved going somewhere and moving actively. It is only relatively recently in terms of human existence that a sedentary day has become a normal day. We are able to obtain food and other necessities with minimal travel, or no travel at all as delivery services have become even more ubiquitous in recent years. We can be entertained from our own homes without leaving the sofa, and our jobs have become increasingly sedentary as many people work sitting at a desk.

We've also seen an increase in disease states associated with a sedentary lifestyle. Heart disease has become the number one cause of death among adult men and women. Some cancers have been increasing in prevalence, particularly those associated with decreased physical activity and increased obesity.[1] Type 2 diabetes mellitus or chronically high blood sugar due to insulin resistance has increased in adults as well as children.

Now, I am not advocating for a preindustrial style of living or the conditions (especially the working conditions) that people faced in past times, but we do need to compensate for this loss of activity in other ways. Many societies have come to that realization in some form or another in the last century, and the idea of exercise as a separate activity specifically for our health began to expand around the middle of the twentieth century. By the 1980s, gyms and fitness centers began cropping up all over major cities. Yet at the same time, the obesity epidemic skyrocketed, and rates of obesity-related disease climbed along with it. Unfortunately, exercise seemed to be marketed mostly as a vanity project. Advertisements stressed the look of a chiseled, attractive body. For some people, this may be motivating. For many

---

[1] National Cancer Institute, "Annual Report."; Biswas et al., "Sedentary Time and Its Association with Risk," 123–132.

others, it seems a luxury not worthy of the time or money required. Many of the popular fitness slogans also stress the idea that pain and difficulty are an important part of the exercise equation, an idea that is certainly not attractive to many people.

So, over the last fifty years, we have seen this incongruous rise in body-shaming along with body positivity. We've seen an increase in available fitness facilities along with increasing rates of heart disease, diabetes, and obesity. We have lost the connection to movement as a natural part of life and turned it into an extra item on an ever-lengthening to-do list. And since exercise seems like an unpleasant activity that we *have* to do, we tend to come up with reasons not to do it, to the detriment of both our physical and mental health.

Even as I was writing this book, the British Journal of Sports Medicine published yet another study examining the benefits of exercise and fitness for our health regardless of weight. This study found that a higher level of cardiovascular fitness (measured in terms of VO_2 max, or a greater amount of oxygen that a person is able to utilize during intense physical activity) is a better marker of our overall health than BMI.[2] The researchers examined several different studies including over 400,000 participants that analyzed these factors, and found that a better VO_2 max lowered a person's risk of both heart disease and mortality from all causes, regardless of their weight category. To put it another way, people who are in good cardiovascular shape or can exercise more have a lower risk of strokes, heart attacks, blood clots, and premature death, whether they are underweight, overweight, or even obese compared with their peers, of all weights, who do not exercise.

I would argue that even more important than living a long life is how we age, or at least how we feel as we age. True, taking less medication and having less frequent visits to hospitals and doctors' offices may be one marker of a good quality of life, but other factors,

---

[2] Weeldreyer et al., "Cardiorespiratory Fitness, Body Mass Index and Mortality," 339–46.

such as a good night's sleep, minimal pain, and a healthy mood are arguably just as, if not even more, important.

When children engage in physical activity, they are not concerned about factors like mortality, controlling blood pressure or blood sugar, or preventing heart disease and dementia. They aren't even concerned with the release of feel-good chemicals that come with exercise. And they are surely not thinking about losing weight. Whereas many grown-ups refer to exercise as something they "should do" and not something they "like to do." We think we should exercise because we want to lose weight or because some mean person like me in a white coat told us it was essential for maintaining our best health. And yes, many of the reasons we "should" exercise are entirely valid. In fact, we definitely do benefit from lower rates of heart disease, diabetes, and high blood pressure. As we grow, we become aware of these other important health concerns and also the fact that our weight is connected to them, but it seems that focusing only on our weight adds to the sense that exercise is a chore rather than a joy, and we become even less inclined to exercise. In contrast, kids simply know that it feels good when they get to move!

Once we start, it *does* feel good to move, largely because of the regulation of our body chemistry that comes with exercise. As our muscles metabolize glucose and lower our blood sugar, our bodies function more optimally. Our cardiovascular system becomes stronger, granting us healthier blood flow throughout our body so that nutrients are carried to our organs, our skin, our muscles, and our joints. Our lungs expand and become more efficient at bringing in oxygen and blowing off carbon dioxide waste products. Our bodies also release endorphins, powerful natural pain killers that literally make our bodies feel better and give our brains a shot of "happy juice." The brain also releases dopamine, the reward chemical that gives us an internal sense of accomplishment. We also find that levels of stress hormones such as cortisol diminish after exercise. And again, for all of these reasons, it *does* feel good to move!

When we change the way that we think about exercise from something that we have to do to something that is natural and even enjoyable, something that will literally help us feel better during and after the process, it becomes a treat instead of a chore. The detriment comes from placing our focus solely on weight loss or weight maintenance, and this for sure makes exercise more like work than fun.

I know a patient, let's call her Sue, who told me that she had not exercised since high school when she had taken part in quite a few sports. She, like many young adult women now, had some features of what we in the medical field call metabolic syndrome (elevated cholesterol and blood sugar levels, slightly elevated blood pressure, and yes, being overweight). But she did not have any compelling disease state that required medication, at least not yet, and therefore nothing serious enough to make her think that it was necessary to make any major lifestyle changes either. Over the course of our conversation, I asked her, "Don't you want to feel good?"

I only know that I asked her this question because she repeated it back to me a couple of months later when she returned for a follow-up visit. She seemed more energetic and generally positive, and she was actually excited to have her labs rechecked, knowing the results would probably be better. She told me that although she had been told previously that her lab work indicated some risk of disease on the horizon, she never felt motivated to make changes to address it. It felt too daunting, and she just thought that she would have to inevitably return to a doctor's office every few months for more bad news until she eventually needed to start medication. It had never dawned on her that she would *feel good now* if she made a few changes right away.

Sue told me that on the day of our initial consultation, she went home thinking "Of course I want to feel good!" and that she was determined to make it happen. She carved out some time in her schedule to start walking at lunch and again after work, at first for about ten minutes at a time. But she eventually built up to thirty-minute walks almost every day during the week and longer walks on weekends, and she announced that she had just started taking yoga classes as well.

I am glad that this phrase spoke to her on that occasion. I'm also disappointed that over several years of doctor's office visits, no one had ever mentioned to her before that one of the benefits of a healthier lifestyle would be an improvement in her overall mood. It took far too long for her to hear that!

Now, Sue was not someone who suffered from a diagnosis of depression or anxiety. She hadn't really even complained of fatigue previously. But she did notice a difference in her energy level and her mood once she started getting outside for walks four to five times a week. And yes, her blood work results did show great improvement in terms of her cholesterol and blood sugar levels, and yes, she had lost a couple of pounds. But the biggest difference I remember seeing in her that day was that she was positively glowing! She reported that she had more energy on a day-to-day basis, and she really looked like someone who felt good.

Another pitfall that comes with focusing too much mental energy on weight loss is that it takes time. We are used to instant results and quick fixes in modern society. Many of us decide we should exercise and hit the gym or the pavement for a few sessions of all-out intensity exercise, which certainly works up a sweat and leaves the muscles sore. But we get frustrated when after a week or two of all that hard work, we have not lost a single pound. In some cases, as we gain muscle, we will initially *add* weight. Oh, the horror! And even though the weight will eventually come off as all that muscle mass boosts our metabolism, many of us would have given up in frustration long before that could happen if our sole focus was on those pesky pounds. I know that Sue would have.

On the other hand, even when the scale hasn't begun to show any benefits from all our hard work, our bodies and minds have already reaped so many meaningful rewards, just as happened for Sue! Even within the first two or three gym sessions or brisk walks, we can feel the brightness of an elevated mood and the peace of a deeper sleep. This is precisely what we should be focusing on! These are the attainable, instant results that will motivate us to *want* to stay active. Who doesn't want to feel good every day?

Instant results are incredibly important to us in this modern age. We see this in the work of the researcher Richard Thaler, who coined the term "present bias," a phenomenon in which human beings prioritize the here and now over long-term rewards.[3] He once observed that when he invited people over to his home for a delicious home-cooked meal, but also set out a bowl of cashews for his guests to snack on while they were waiting, many of his guests enjoyed the cashews even though they knew that a full meal was coming, even to the detriment of their appetite when the food arrived. The idea of the future delicious food was no match for the simple nuts that were already present.

Similar studies have been conducted where participants, in some cases young children, were offered a sweet treat such as a marshmallow. They were told that they could have the treat right in front of them now, or, if they waited a set length of time (fifteen minutes, for example), they could have two marshmallows.[4] The researchers surmised that this experiment in children offered some insight into which personalities exhibited more self-control, but the fact remains that the majority of the participants chose the immediate, smaller reward over the larger reward that they would have to wait for. Our natural inclination is to want results, rewards, or satisfaction immediately, even if the immediate satisfaction is substandard.

Thaler's original studies and these other later experiments often focused on tangible goods, such as the food in the examples above, but the concept can also apply to behaviors. Most of us still tend to prefer a smaller, faster reward over a larger reward that requires waiting. This is part of why it is easy to value the pleasure of cozying up on the couch while watching television over the abstract idea that we might be healthier in a few months if we were to get up and

---

[3] Thaler, *Misbehaving*.
[4] Mischel, *The Marshmallow Test: Mastering Self-Control*.

take a walk. We know that exercise reduces the chance that we will have a stroke or heart attack later in life, but so often that feels like something we can deal with later.

Too often, those habits that we know we should do fall into categories that offer a future reward. What makes them difficult is that these future rewards are neither tangible enough nor immediate enough to really motivate the behavior needed right now to achieve that future reward.

We can use this psychology to our advantage if we shift the focus away from the long-term benefits that we are looking to gain and replace that focus on the more instantaneous gratification of a better night's sleep or a brightened mood. When we refocus the emphasis of our physical activity away from the results that we hope to see in several months' time to a present reward, such as having more energy today, it becomes much easier to enjoy.

Weight loss takes a long time, for many people far too long to be a consistently motivating goal. The reason for that is that the excess weight we want to shed, or fat cells, are stored energy to our bodies. We do need a certain amount of stored energy for our bodies to function. Otherwise, we would not be able to sleep through the night or fast for long periods, even a few hours between meals as our organs, especially our brain, require a constant supply of energy even at rest. We measure this stored energy in terms of potential, or in calories, which most people are familiar with. The number of calories (actually kilocalories, or "kcals," to be precise) in one pound of body fat tissue is equal to about 3,500 kcal. This means that in order to lose one pound of body fat in one week, we would have to run an energy deficit of (or use up an extra) 3,500 calories, which breaks down into about five hundred calories per day. Consider that most adults' resting metabolism (the amount of energy burned on any given day at rest) averages between 1,500 to 2,000 calories per day. This means that in order to lose one pound of body fat, a healthy adult would have to either consume five hundred calories less than their resting metabolism (about 1,000 to 1,500 calories) every day for one week. Or we would have to utilize or "burn" an extra five hundred calories in the form of work or movement (aka exercise), or do some combination of the two. And that still adds up to only losing one pound in one week. For most of us, this is a lot of work for seemingly little reward. No wonder most of us give up in frustration after seven hard days of fighting cravings and exercising intensely, only to find that the dial on the scale is in roughly the same place it was before! Now, true, in the long run, this does add up. So if you were to maintain these efforts over the course of, say, three months, you would have indeed lost twelve to fifteen pounds, or thereabouts depending on how strictly you maintained these activities every day.

Those at a larger body mass to begin with may see results faster since, at first, their resting metabolism is higher just as a function of having more body mass. But as the body mass declines, so does the resting metabolism, because a smaller body utilizes less energy for the basic functions that sustain life, and I find that, especially for my patients in this category, the desire to maintain the healthy habits developed at the beginning of their weight loss efforts depends heavily on whether they have found enjoyment in these healthy habits for reasons other than weight loss.

In Sue's case, she did eventually lose a bit of body weight, and her cholesterol and blood sugar levels improved dramatically, allowing her to avoid medication for these concerns and likely prevent an impending heart attack or stroke later in life. But as she would tell you, none of that seems important on the day-to-day basis in between our periodic check-ins in the clinic. What is important to her now, as it well should be, is that she *feels good*!

CHAPTER 3

Neurochemicals

Exercise is a powerful treatment for our mental health. Most people will notice after some physical activity that they feel a sense of calm, or accomplishment, or even euphoria. There are several explanations for this, and over recent years, researchers have debated the importance of certain "feel-good chemicals" over others, but the fact remains that there are several natural chemicals and processes that contribute to our feeling better after exercise. Exercise helps our bodies to release powerful chemicals such as endorphins, enkephalins, dopamine, and serotonin, while reducing levels of stress chemicals such as cortisol and adrenaline. These substances are all natural compounds that serve an important function in our bodies, whether or not we are aware of them. They help us to move efficiently, recover more easily, and handle outside stressors.

For most of human history, the stressors we had to deal with involved situations such as escaping danger or finding food, both of which required activity. We would have *had* to move to run away from a predator or fight off an attacker, whether it be human or animal. And we had to walk or run to find food and bring it back to our home or community. Our ability to release adrenaline along with a short burst of cortisol meant that we could go farther and faster without getting tired. Adrenaline helps to increase the heart rate, open up the lungs, expand our field of vision, and divert blood flow toward the working muscles. We would also produce enkephalins during these activities so that we could continue to run or climb or fight without feeling pain or becoming emotionally overwhelmed at the danger we were in.

The stressors we face in modern society are much different. We get stuck in traffic or have to deal with coworkers, bosses, and customers who make us uncomfortable or irritable at work. Plus, we're constantly hearing news about all the worrisome or dangerous events in the world. Our bodies release the same adrenaline that we would have needed in past times of stress, but without the movement to utilize that adrenaline, we instead end up feeling wired and anxious. We can sense the rapid heartbeat and increased breath rate, but we cannot utilize these responses as they are meant to be used, that is to move quickly and get out of danger. Our vision can become blurry and extra sensitive to light, causing headaches. And without movement, we do not produce the increased endorphins to tolerate the mental and emotional part of that stress, or subdue the physical pain that is ramped up by it. So we simply feel on edge. However, scheduling some movement into our day helps us to balance these chemicals. Several studies have examined the effects of exercise on the measurable levels of these compounds, and we have found that exercise, especially regular and recurrent exercise, helps us to reset and maintain optimal balance.

ENDORPHINS / ENKEPHALINS

Endorphins and enkephalins are peptide chemicals (large proteins) made by our bodies. They are also known as "endogenous opioids," meaning they have a similar effect to opioid drugs on reducing pain in our bodies, but unlike medications or drugs, they are "endogenous," meaning that they are produced inside our own selves naturally.

These chemicals are produced in higher amounts when we engage in physical activity, an effect demonstrated in many studies over the last thirty years.[5] The main difference between endorphins and enkephalins for the purpose of this discussion is that, in general, enkephalins bind to the spinal cord, whereas endorphins are found to bind to certain areas of the brain. This is a bit of an overgeneralization, but for the purposes of this discussion, we will consider these chemicals as a group with similar function and purpose. Both of these substances have powerful pain-killing properties similar to narcotic or opioid medications, but without so many of the terrible side effects associated with opioid drugs. Endorphins not only work on the receptors in our brains to relieve pain, but they have also been thought to increase our sense of happiness as well as go on to trigger the release of other mood-boosting chemicals such as dopamine, which we will discuss more in a moment. For many years, scientists and clinicians have believed that endorphins were the chemicals most responsible for the euphoric sensation people often feel after exercise, sometimes referred to as the "runner's high." We now know that several other chemicals also play a role in this sense of euphoria, but endorphins still get most of the credit among athletic circles.

Endorphins and enkephalins also affect other processes and chemicals in our bodies that contribute to our sense of elation and decrease our sense of pain. A study from Harvard Medical School showed that enkephalins help to decrease another peptide chemical that our bodies produce called substance P.[6] Substance P is a neurotransmitter (chemical that signals to the brain) mostly responsible for triggering pain, but it is also involved in neuroinflammation, nausea and vomiting, gastrointestinal distress, and according to some recent studies, emotional pain as well.[7] We now know that when enkephalin is released, it binds to nerve cells and prevents certain kinds of these

---

[5] Francis, "The Role of Endorphins in Exercise," 169–73.
[6] Mudge et al., "Enkephalin Inhibits Release of Substance P," 526–30.
[7] Ebner et al., "Substance P in the Medial Amygdala," 4280–5.

cells from releasing too much substance P, leading to lower levels of this chemical and the unpleasant effects associated with it. It literally stops the pain signal from being released!

Individuals with higher levels of endorphins and enkephalins are noted to tolerate higher amounts of physical pain as well as emotional stress. This makes sense if you think about how our bodies were made to react to stress from early on in our human existence. We would be able to run away from danger without feeling pain from the act of running, and we could block out the emotional stress that might come from the thought that someone or something is chasing us. The endorphin/enkephalin release allowed us to keep going, to escape harm and feel good about it, and to avoid discomfort along the way. We can see how this phenomenon would be helpful in a natural setting, but we can also use it to our advantage in our present daily lives. Since we know that exercise increases our endorphin and enkephalin levels, and we know that higher levels help us to handle emotional stress, we can see how going for a walk or riding a bike in the morning can help us handle a stressful meeting in the afternoon or feel calmer while sitting in a traffic jam on the way home. When we have moved our bodies, we can literally tolerate these stressors more easily.

DOPAMINE

As I mentioned a moment ago, the increase in endorphins also helps to trigger the release of other chemicals. One of these chemicals is dopamine. Dopamine is often referred to as the chemical of desire, but it's more like the chemical of fixation. We get repeated moments of dopamine release when we engage in certain activities that the brain has deemed necessary for survival: eating food, spending time with friends and family, having sex, watching something entertaining, or even playing a game or scrolling social media. Dopamine helps us form connections to these activities and makes us crave them. Any parent who has tried to take away a video game device or turn off the television in front of a child can attest to the powerful hold dopamine surges have over the brain. And while some activities that stimulate dopamine leave us feeling tired or worn out afterward (too much candy or screen time for instance), dopamine can also be increased by activities that leave us feeling better after the fact. One such activity is exercise.

Thankfully for us, dopamine is shown to remain increased in people who exercise regularly. This is partially because some of the exercise endorphins trigger dopamine releases in other centers of the brain. But even more profoundly, the amount of dopamine that the brain releases will increase over time as exercise becomes a regular habit.[8] Like many parts of the body, the more you use it, the stronger and/or larger it becomes. So over time, we see that exercise actually increases the size and structure of the reward center of the brain, leading to higher circulating levels of dopamine as well as more available receptors for that dopamine to attach to. In short, the brain is, at baseline, primed to make and receive more dopamine and to experience this pleasure more easily when exercise becomes a regular part of our routine.

This increase in dopamine is particularly important to aging adults, since in normal aging, dopamine receptors decline gradually, up to 14 percent with each decade, according to some models.[9] The decline in dopamine and in dopamine receptors likely leads to higher rates of depression among older adults. Exercise in our older population can not only prevent, but actually reverse this decline in dopamine receptors, making physical activity particularly important for aging adults. For our younger adults, maximizing your potential brain health early in life offers long-lasting benefits as we optimize the dopamine-producing and -receiving cells, so we enter into our later years with a stronger system. And of course, this dopamine boost also helps us feel better immediately.

---

[8] Bastioli et al., "Voluntary Exercise Boosts Striatal Dopamine Release," 4725–36.
[9] Karrer, "Reduced Dopamine Receptors," 36–46.

Dopamine also plays a role in cravings or addictions. In fact, it is the main chemical that we focus on with medications to help our patients who struggle with addiction. By increasing baseline dopamine levels, we are able to help patients quit smoking, for example. It seems that having a higher, steadier stream of dopamine helps to minimize the cravings for things that we usually turn to in order to obtain that quick dopamine jolt. So, taking a regular walk or trip to the gym may also help us to curb or quit these less desirable habits while establishing healthy ones. And as our bodies begin to associate exercise with an increase in dopamine, we come to look forward to physical activity, or even crave it!

We also utilize dopamine-boosting medication to help with mood and focus, including in the treatment of ADHD and depression. This chemical's role in our attention span and its clear response to exercise may be a large part of the reason that our patients who struggle with ADHD feel and perform better after physical exertion. I remember my son's pediatrician recommending at the age of six or seven that he exercise before school to help with his attention span, and it has helped! Even now, years later, I can see a huge difference in both of my children's behavior and focus on days when they have exercised versus when they have not. Some days we are able to get in a longer walk or a bit of jogging, but some mornings when we're pressed for time, we'll at least do some jumping jacks and crunches, and this couple of minutes seems to make a big difference for them. Plus, it's a fun way to start the day!

In short, we know the importance of dopamine, and we know that exercise gives us both a momentary boost and a more robust dopamine-producing and -receiving system in the long term. If dopamine was the only chemical affected by exercise, this alone would be a terrific benefit. But as we've seen, the systems and benefits are many.

SEROTONIN

Exercise also increases our serotonin levels, thought to be the single most important neurochemical in regulating our mood as well as our sleep cycle. Serotonin is so important, in fact, that most of our medications aimed at treating depression and anxiety are primarily targeted at increasing circulating serotonin levels.

Serotonin is yet another chemical considered to be a neurotransmitter, or something that sends signals throughout the brain. Certain areas of the brain and other nerves are responsible for producing this chemical, and other areas of the brain and nervous system have receptors, basically keyholes, that serotonin molecules fit into. These receptors function as off and on switches for several activities in the brain. In the case of serotonin, there are many different receptors with different functions, so serotonin levels can affect several different functions in the brain, ultimately influencing mood, digestion, libido, appetite, and more. Serotonin also stimulates areas of the brain that control our sleep-wake cycles. It can both wake us up and be converted into melatonin, which is necessary for inducing sleep. When serotonin levels are in an ideal range, we tend to feel calmer, more focused, and emotionally stable, and we sleep more deeply. On the contrary, when serotonin levels are abnormally low, we find that people are more prone to anxiety or excessive worry, fitful sleep, obsessive behaviors like picking, scratching, or compulsive cleaning, and cravings for substances like sugar, salt, and alcohol. I also observe that irritability is one of the most common symptoms of both depression and anxiety that my patients report. When our serotonin levels are low, we are less able to handle daily stressors without feeling serious tension, even rage.

One of my patients who complained of feeling stressed reported that she became extremely annoyed with people so easily that a minor infraction would send her into mental frenzy. We discussed several methods to help her balance these emotions, including medication and therapy, as well as adding a daily walk before work.

When she returned for a follow-up, she reported back that "yeah, the annoying guy at work is still annoying, but I no longer want to throw my chair at him!" Success! We can't control all the irritations that come our way over the course of the day, but when our brain chemistry, particularly serotonin, is in better balance, we can handle those stressors more easily. Again, for some people, this may require medication, but with or without medical treatment, we can get a major boost from some daily activity.

Serotonin also plays a major role in our sleep-wake cycle. I cannot even begin to count the number of patients I see who complain of having poor sleep. And while there are many medications available to help induce or prolong sleep, they all have their downsides, including the fact that for some people, they simply don't work, and that for many others, they still feel tired and foggy the following day. Another major issue is that most of our sleep medications create dependency to the extent that after taking them for some time, our patients find that they cannot fall asleep without them.

In addition to and sometimes in place of medications, we often discuss certain behavior changes, collectively called "sleep hygiene," to help address sleep difficulties. It is no surprise that one of the major tenets of sleep hygiene is to include some exercise during the day. Some sleep hygiene literature stresses the timing of exercise as well, so that the body has the optimal amount of time to relax after exertion, but we see that exercise throughout the waking hours at any time will help bring on a good night's sleep the following evening. And even better, this improves with the frequency of exercise, likely due, at least in part, to the improved function of the parts of the serotonin system involved in regulating the sleep-wake cycle. And the serotonin system, like other parts of the brain and nervous system, develops and strengthens over time with regular use.

Serotonin also plays an important role in digestion. In recent years, we have come to learn more about the so-called "gut-brain axis." Serotonin is now known to help stimulate digestion. In fact, low levels of serotonin are associated with higher incidence of constipation and irritable bowel syndrome, or IBS.[10]

Serotonin also controls the nausea centers in the gastrointestinal tract, and it influences the appetite, helping us to feel full. This may be one reason why people suffering from depression tend to either overeat or lose their appetite in compensation for their mood. In addition to affecting the appetite, serotonin affects the digestion process itself, literally helping to keep the gastrointestinal tract muscles moving in sequence, which keeps the gut more regular. This helps us avoid painful conditions like constipation and cramps. Understanding serotonin's role in our gut health also explains, at least in part, why these symptoms are seen more frequently in people who suffer from depression.

Several studies over the past four decades have shown that exercise increases the speed and activity of serotonin neurons, meaning that physical activity increases the production and release of the chemical serotonin. At this point, there are almost too many studies to point to individually, and several of them are summed up nicely in an editorial in the *Journal of Psychiatry and Neuroscience*, entitled "How to Increase Serotonin in the Human Brain Without Drugs,"[11] written by Dr. Simon Young. As a side note, Dr. Young also discusses several studies that found that exposure to bright light also positively affects or increases serotonin levels, which makes sense as light therapy is part of the standard treatment for seasonal depression. Light therapy is also being used now for nonseasonal depression and some related conditions such as premenstrual dysphoric disorder. So when we exercise outdoors, or even in a brightly lit gym or studio, the effect on our mood is even more powerful.

Now, there are certain medical conditions and instances when treatment with serotonin-boosting medication is necessary, and I will not suggest that spending time outdoors or exercising will

---

[10] Vahora et al., "Serotonin Level Fluctuation," e9871.
[11] Young, "How to Increase Serotonin," 394–9.

completely replace treatment for these patients. But still, exercise and outdoor activity should be considered an important part of the treatment plan. And for many of us who suffer the effects of an occasional slump in serotonin levels, exercise can help us maximize this important, natural neurochemical and feel our best.

NEUROPEPTIDE Y

Another important neurochemical that is influenced by exercise and slightly newer to scientific discussion is neuropeptide Y (NPY). Don't be scared by the name. NPY literally means "brain-protein Y." It is produced in the brain and circulated throughout the nervous system, but it's mostly concentrated in areas of the brain called the hippocampus and the amygdala.[12] Although NPY wasn't even discovered until 1982, we now know that it is one of the most abundant proteins in the nervous system. Recent research demonstrates a dramatic increase in the production of NPY with exercise, particularly with aerobic exercise.[13]

Researchers have also found that higher levels of NPY correlate with lower anxiety responses in both animals and humans.[14] In fact, the amygdala itself is more highly active in people who suffer from chronic anxiety or post-traumatic stress disorder, but this activity is somehow calmed down by an increase in neuropeptide Y.[15] Several scientists now credit NPY as the primary source of runner's high, given its strong effects on decreasing anxiety and depression symptoms. I have heard researchers claim that the effect of neuropeptide Y may be even stronger than that of endorphins. I

---

[12] Eaton et al., "Relevance of Neuropeptide Y," 1645–59.
[13] Kienast et al., "Neuropeptide Y – Its Role in Human Performance," 10032.
[14] Brené et al., "Running is Rewarding and Antidepressive," 136–140.
[15] Eaton et al., "Relevance of Neuropeptide Y," 1645–59.

tend to believe that it is a combination of several factors, but either way, we know this chemical is one of them!

Neuropeptide Y also helps tremendously with sleep, including reducing the amount of time it takes to fall asleep and the ability to stay asleep. The influence of this chemical on our circadian rhythm actually rivals the effect of natural light, long thought to have the most important influence on our sleep. This is yet another way (in addition to serotonin mentioned earlier) in which exercise encourages restful, deep, and prolonged sleep. I sometimes remind myself after a late night or an evening when I did not sleep well that despite how tired I may feel in the very early hours of the morning, getting in a quick jog or some resistance training before work will help me sleep better the following night, and it works every time.

We are still learning more about neuropeptide Y, but we already know without a doubt that this peptide has much to offer our sense of well-being, and that we have the ability to boost it through aerobic activity.

ENDOCANNABINOID

The last decade has seen a steep rise in the popularity of products aimed at influencing the cannabinoid system, namely CBD products, which have been popping up in pharmacies, beauty shops, grocery stores, and even CBD specialty markets. These products have a compelling effect on sleep, pain relief, relaxation, and calm. They work in our bodies by triggering specially programmed receptors, similar to how narcotic pain medications mimic endorphins in our bodies and trigger pain-blocking opioid receptors. Human beings make two different main types of chemicals that scientists have dubbed "endocannabinoids," which bind to just under a dozen different receptors. These receptors generally function as either mood regulators or pain regulators, and they are another likely contributor to exercise-induced euphoria, or runner's high. Interestingly, the endocannabinoids that our bodies produce also help aid our memory, whereas cannabinoid medications or drugs tend to cause mental impairment.

Some of these receptors also have an effect on stimulating our appetite. In fact, the cannabinoid system's effect on appetite was once thought to be the key to a possible weight loss medication, and this demonstrates another example of people sacrificing their overall health in the name of weight. The medication was aimed at blocking the cannabinoid receptors in the brain, and it did work to decrease appetite. However, after only a short time on the market, it was recalled on an emergency basis for causing suicidal thoughts in people who took it. In the end, this terrible and unintentional consequence did reveal how important the endocannabinoid system is in regulating our emotional well-being.

Recent research done at Wayne University has shown that exercise consistently increases the body's endocannabinoids.[16] This effect was observed across different types of exercise including running, swimming, and weight lifting, but was most noticeable with moderate- to high-intensity aerobic activity that elevated the heart rate for at least thirty minutes.

These chemicals, produced naturally by our own bodies, offer us a sense of happiness, calm, relaxation, and pain relief. They are essentially the brain's reward to the body for accomplishing the task of movement. Again, this makes sense from a survival standpoint. Movement means survival—it means we're finding food or locating a group to belong to and travel with. Movement also means setting up a living space, caring for children, and, yes, engaging in procreation. These are all necessary for human survival, and they all require movement, or at least they did for most of human history. Our brains have spent thousands of years surviving in this way, creating

---

[16] Marusak, "The 'Runner's High.'"

these "way-to-go" chemicals to reward our bodies for moving, and therefore surviving. So yet again, it feels good to move!

CORTISOL

Exercise also lowers levels of cortisol, sometimes called the stress hormone. In recent years, I've noticed that more of my patients have become familiar with this hormone in our bodies, likely as many have realized the effects of prolonged stress on their own health and sense of well-being. Cortisol in short bursts or small doses can actually be helpful, even essential to our bodies. Cortisol increases sugars (glucose) in the bloodstream, enhances the brain's use of that glucose, and increases the body's ability to repair tissues such as muscles. These functions would be essential in a state of danger. Combined with adrenaline, which raises the heart rate and narrows blood vessels in order to direct blood to the working parts of the body, this allows the body to move quickly and with greater strength. Cortisol also curbs functions that would not be essential in a fight-or-flight situation, so it slows down digestion and suppresses the immune system, the reproductive system, and physical growth. This response is usually temporary, and cortisol levels will usually return to normal once a threat has passed, so the immune system will return to full function, blood sugar will return to normal, and growth and repair will resume. However, chronic stress, something we face often in modern society, does not dissipate in the same way that these historical dangers would have.

There are two opposing sides to our nervous system. The sympathetic nervous system, often referred to as "fight or flight," kicks in to deal with stressors. Its counterpart, the parasympathetic nervous system, or "rest and digest," predominates when we want to engage in activities such as sleeping, eating, and even intercourse.

But in conditions of chronic stress, the sympathetic nervous system remains activated, while the counterbalancing parasympathetic system remains suppressed. As a result our cortisol levels increase in the long term. This increases our risk for weight gain, illness due to a weakened immune system, chronically elevated blood pressure and blood sugar, anxiety and depression, digestive problems, difficulty sleeping, and muscle pain. If these symptoms sound familiar, you may already be suffering from chronically elevated cortisol levels. The good news is that you have the ability to bring them down!

When we exercise, especially at a high intensity, our bodies activate the sympathetic nervous system, causing an initial increase in adrenaline and, yes, in cortisol as well. However, research has shown that about thirty minutes after starting exercise, the cortisol levels begin to drop, and they reach a low point about thirty minutes after exercise has ended.[17]

Several studies have also shown that individuals who exercise frequently maintain lower baseline levels of cortisol,[18] countering the common trend toward chronically elevated cortisol levels that we see in our sedentary population. This is not to say that people who exercise do not encounter chronic stress, but their bodies are better equipped to handle it. With exercise, our bodies are able to experience temporary, short-term bursts of fight or flight, then return to long periods of rest and digest, partially thanks to a natural rise and fall in cortisol along with its partner chemicals in the nervous system, which we will discuss next. This not only helps to keep our blood sugar and blood pressure under control, as well as prevent fatty tissue from accumulating around our midsection, but it also helps us feel calmer. This decline in cortisol then allows the immune system to function more effectively and allows our bodies to process nutrients and repair injuries so that we experience less pain and keep moving.

---

[17] Rudolph et al., "Cortisol and Affective Responses to Exercise," 122–8.
[18] De Nys et al., "The Effects of Physical Activity," 105843.

ADRENALINE

Adrenaline, also called epinephrine, and noradrenaline, or norepinephrine, are the primary compounds used by our autonomic nervous system, the system that controls the automatic functions in our body like heart rate, breathing, vision, and digestion—essentially things that function without us having to think about it.

Similar to cortisol, our bodies are made to release adrenaline in response to anything that is perceived as a threat, activating the components of the sympathetic nervous system, which include a faster heart rate, quicker breathing, dilated pupils, sweating, and constricted or narrowed blood vessels. We also experience an extra release of adrenaline when we exercise, and that adrenaline helps to raise our heart rate and breathing rate, allowing the body to take in more oxygen and get it back out to the working muscles more efficiently. Adrenaline activates our sweat glands to produce sweat so that we do not overheat, and it narrows our blood vessels to push blood to the working muscles.

Modern stressors also trigger an increase in adrenaline, and when we experience those stressors in a sedentary condition (like sitting in traffic or at a computer reading an alarming email), we experience the rapid heartbeat, shallow breathing, increased sweating, and even tunnel vision—and it feels terrible! For those who suffer from repeated adrenaline rushes and experience these symptoms often, the best way to get rid of that excess adrenaline is of course to use it up through movement. Exercise utilizes adrenaline for its intended purpose: to help us move. As movement burns it off as fuel for the fight-or-flight response, we experience lower levels of this chemical at rest. Our bodies are constantly at work to maintain a balance between the two opposing sides of our autonomic nervous system, so once we have engaged the sympathetic system and utilized the adrenaline provided, our bodies shift into a predominantly parasympathetic state more readily, allowing us to rest and recover.

For many of my patients who suffer from recurrent panic attacks, exercise is a key component of their treatment plan, and not just because going out for a walk or to a yoga class helps to provide stress relief in that moment. The chemical balance that exercise induces lasts long after the exercise session is finished.

People who suffer from panic attacks typically experience them, as they describe it, "out of nowhere." The attacks, which are essentially adrenaline rushes gone rogue, seem to occur while sitting and watching TV, driving somewhere familiar, or getting ready for bed. It seems to be those occasions that feel fairly simple and automatic—where the brain is on autopilot, conscious mental activity is quiet, and the subconscious background chatter dominates—that the most ferocious panic attacks take hold. It is in these moments that the primal part of our brains seems to remember that we have suppressed feelings of stress earlier in the day, and there is a flood of adrenaline still waiting to be released. So bam! Here it is. And it not only feels terrible physically, but it can be really emotionally scary.

We are still not exactly sure why these happen or why some people are more prone to them than others, but we do know that people who exercise more often are less likely to suffer from panic attacks and anxiety symptoms in general. This is at least partially due to a lower baseline level of adrenaline in people who exercise regularly. It may also have something to do with an improved balance of the other neurochemicals mentioned earlier, like serotonin and endorphins or a combination of all of the above. A balanced combination of all these chemicals serves as powerful mental health medicine through multiple channels.

To summarize, exercise increases our feel-good chemicals like dopamine, serotonin, endorphins, enkephalins, endocannabinoids, and neuropeptide Y, and it reduces our long-term build-up of chemicals like cortisol and adrenaline. What does all this chemical soup mean for you? Most importantly, by exercising, you will *feel better*, and it is not simply because you know you have done something healthy for yourself when you complete a walk, exercise class, or session at the gym. There are actual chemical rewards released in your brain and body that literally boost your mood, make it easier to focus, reduce symptoms of panic and anxiety, and help you sleep better at night. And you can access this treatment whenever and however you like. The key is just to start moving!

CHAPTER 4

Hormones

One of the requests I hear most often in the clinic is "can you check my hormones?" I am astounded at how frequently patients come in for symptoms such as fatigue or a depressed mood and their first conclusion is that their sex hormones must be out of whack. My patients, like the general population, have become increasingly aware of the effects of the balance (or imbalance) in our testosterone, estrogen, and progesterone levels. While there are many medical conditions that cause abnormal levels of these hormones (either too low or too high), and these conditions may need treatment, often these hormones are near the upper or lower limits of normal, but still technically normal. However, patients may feel some of the effects of this less-than-ideal balance. Many of these mild imbalances may be corrected or at least helped by lifestyle changes rather than or in addition to hormonal medications, which, like all medications, come with some potential risks and side effects. And as we have already seen, many of the symptoms that people attribute to low hormone levels, such as fatigue, weight change, low libido, irregular cycles, and moodiness, may also be due to an imbalance of the other chemicals we have already discussed. We already know that exercise helps balance these chemicals, and the good news for anyone who is concerned about their hormone levels is that exercise, both endurance (or cardiovascular exercise) and resistance (or weight training exercise), has been shown to regulate circulating levels of hormones.

One of the conditions associated with hormone imbalance that we see most often is a condition known as polycystic ovarian syndrome (or PCOS), a very common though difficult-to-treat condition. In women who suffer from PCOS, the ovaries produce excessive amounts of hormones such as estrogen and androgens, a group of sex hormones, including testosterone, commonly associated with male characteristics. This imbalance can lead to irregular cycles, problems with acne, male-pattern hair loss on the scalp, unwanted hair on the face and body, and low fertility. Women with PCOS are also at increased risk for insulin resistance, leading to prediabetes or diabetes, as well as cardiovascular disease, fatty liver, and mood disorders such as anxiety and depression.

The insulin resistance associated with PCOS creates a vicious cycle whereby body fat increases in the form of fat cells, or what we call adipose tissue. Frustratingly, these fat cells further increase androgen hormones in women, making PCOS symptoms worse. For this reason, weight loss, diet, and exercise have long been part of the treatment for women with PCOS, but weight loss seems particularly difficult for women with this condition, furthering the frustration for many of my patients who battle this syndrome. This is one condition in particular where I find that focusing on the function of exercise rather than weight loss is key.

A meta-analysis published in 2020 in the *Journal of Kinesiology* examined the effects of exercise in women with PCOS.[19] The analysis found that not only did cardio and resistance training help to normalize androgen levels for these women, but even low-impact exercise practices such as yoga also imparted some improvement in hormone levels and symptoms, and this effect was noted whether or not the women in these studies lost weight. So yet again, whether or not the pounds on the scale showed any change, these women achieved noticeable changes in their bodies at a chemical level, not to mention

---

[19] Shele et al., "Effects of Exercise on Hormones," 35.

the meaningful improvement in terms of hair pattern, skin condition, cycle regularity, and mood! Not surprisingly, vigorous exercise decreased insulin resistance by the greatest amount, but even mild- to moderate-intensity exercise made a difference. And the decrease in insulin resistance was even seen after only one session of exercise!

In a study published by *Breast Cancer Research*, exercise has also been shown to decrease total androgen levels in women without polycystic ovarian syndrome and significantly reduce the risk of estrogen-receptor-positive breast cancers.[20] In this study, twenty-three different randomized controlled trials were analyzed to examine the effects of exercise on either free or total estradiol (estrogen) levels. The researchers reported a significant decrease in estradiol in the study participants who exercised. They also found that physical activity reduced free-testosterone levels in the women and increased a protein called sex hormone binding globulin (SHBG), which is essential for moving these androgen hormones through the body.

Now I would not suggest that all cancers can be cured by a daily walk, but it is worth noting that a sedentary lifestyle is considered a risk factor for several types of cancers, including breast and colon cancers. There has been a dramatic increase in several of these types of cancers in correlation with our increasingly sedentary lifestyles over the last several decades. Exercise is thought to reduce the risk of several types of cancer through both lowering inflammatory body fat and also decreasing hormone and chemical levels that are known to increase the incidence of these cancers.

Interestingly, while routine exercise lowered or normalized testosterone levels in women, physical activity, especially resistance training exercise, has been shown to *increase* testosterone levels in men. Men with low testosterone levels may experience decreased libido (sex drive), difficulty with getting or maintaining an erection during sex, decreased muscle and bone mass, difficulty sleeping, depressed mood, fatigue, and of course increase in body fat. In both

---

[20] Ennour-Idrissi et al., "Effect of Physical Activity on Sex Hormones," 139.

men and women, adipose tissue (or fat cells) contain enzymes that convert testosterone into estrogen. So as we gain weight, testosterone levels become lower and lower while estrogen levels rise, in men as well as women. Just as PCOS can create a frustrating cycle of weight gain and insulin resistance with a further tendency toward more weight gain in women, low testosterone levels in men often create an upsetting trend toward fatigue, low muscle mass, and further weight gain. Thankfully, exercise can help reverse this trend, partially through reducing fatty tissue, and thereby reducing the breakdown of testosterone into estrogen, but also through the act of exercise alone. Even small changes in activity levels can increase muscle mass, which further helps to increase testosterone levels and decrease the occurrence of testosterone converting into estrogen.

In both sexes, testosterone levels tend to peak fifteen minutes after exercise, which is necessary for muscle growth and repair. Our bodies need this temporary spike because testosterone aids the body in converting amino acids into larger proteins that the muscles can utilize to rebuild themselves. Here again, the body is very good at giving itself what it needs to heal given the appropriate triggers. So it makes sense that our bodies are essentially wired to deliver this testosterone boost right when we need it for repair and recovery. Testosterone also helps to counteract some of the effects of cortisol and prevents the breakdown of other proteins in the body. In the long term, as our bodies increase muscle mass and burn fat cells, the testosterone levels remain higher, especially in men, since men's bodies produce testosterone from two sources (the testicles and adrenal glands), compared to women, who receive testosterone almost solely from the adrenal glands. Other factors, such as nutrition, sleep, and alcohol also have an impact on testosterone levels, so exercise should be considered one lifestyle factor of many for men who want to naturally increase their testosterone levels. But overall, exercise is a powerful factor indeed, in both the immediate and the long term.

Probably the most common hormone-driven condition that my

female patients complain about are the symptoms associated with menopause. For women in menopause, weight gain seems particularly frustrating. As our hormones decline in the fifth and sixth decades of life, we lose not only our previous levels of estrogen and progesterone, but also our testosterone, which contributes to a decrease in muscle mass, affecting not only our strength and physical appearance, but also our resting metabolism! Weight-bearing exercise (strength training) counters this by increasing muscle mass and boosting our androgen hormones (just as it does in men), allowing us to continue to build more muscle, which maximizes our metabolism throughout the day. So we burn more calories, even at rest.

For women in menopause, bone density loss is another major concern, and for decades, the primary advice for building and maintaining bone density has included a healthy diet that includes plenty of calcium and vitamin D as well as a hefty amount of weight-bearing exercise. As we push and pull with our muscles, they in turn apply some physical stress or force to the bones where they connect, and the body responds to these repeated forces by building stronger, more dense bones, preventing and even reversing conditions like osteopenia and osteoporosis, conditions which indicate that the bones are more likely to fracture. While this may seem like an abstract health benefit that takes a long time to achieve and feel too intangible to provide motivation now, the reality of osteoporosis is that people, especially women, can suffer from devastating and painful fractures (broken hips, wrists, or vertebrae). The spine can fracture slowly over time, leading to a cumbersome rounding of the spinal posture and incredibly debilitating back pain. Weight-bearing exercise such as weight lifting, Pilates, yoga, HIIT, and others increases the density of our bones and prevents this kind of painful event from happening, which keeps us feeling good and moving easily.

Another common complaint that I hear from my patients facing menopause is, of course, the hot flashes. We know that during an exercise session, we are likely to get hot and sweaty, but who wants to experience random flashes of heat and sweat, seemingly out of nowhere? And of course, hot flashes happen at either the most embarrassing times possible or, even worse, just in time to wake you from sleep. Thankfully, exercise has been shown to decrease the basal body temperature of women in perimenopause and menopause,[21] which makes sense as we know that exercise also lowers the basal body temperature of men and nonmenopausal women. This study showed that not only did the core temperature adjust, but the body's ability to regulate both blood flow to the skin and sweat gland activity also improved. In fact, the women in this study reported 60 percent fewer hot flashes! So let's sweat it out at the gym instead of in our bedsheets!

For men with low testosterone, or "low-T syndrome," women with polycystic ovarian syndrome, or women with menopausal symptoms, there are hormone medications that medical providers prescribe to help our patients manage their symptoms. But as with all medications, there are risks associated with them, including blood clots, changes in mood, and increased cancer risks. Moreover, the medications are seldom effective at addressing every symptom associated with these conditions. Exercise, on the other hand, not only helps our patients balance hormone levels and feel better, but it is also relatively side-effect free.

---

[21] Bailey et al., "Frequency of Menopausal Hot Flushes," 708–18.

CHAPTER 5

Digestion

Many of us take our digestive system for granted until it doesn't function well for any length of time. It really is a complex and underappreciated system—underappreciated, that is, until it malfunctions and we experience bloating, fatigue, and even physical pain.

First, let's talk about normal digestion and gut health. Gastrointestinal function involves several key processes that work together to digest food, absorb nutrients, and eliminate waste. Food and liquid enters through the mouth, where the digestive process begins as the contents are chewed and mixed with saliva, which contains enzymes that help break down the nutrients that can be absorbed and used later. Food then travels through the esophagus to the stomach, where it mixes with highly acidic gastric juices (hence the pain of acid reflux when this acid escapes the stomach and gets back up into the esophagus behind the breastbone). These acidic juices liquify and sterilize the incoming food, then move it into the small intestine, where even more digestive enzymes are added thanks to delivery from the pancreas and liver. All these enzymes break the nutrients down so that they can start to be absorbed through the lining of the small intestine into the bloodstream.

I remember being amazed in anatomy class at how my blood

vessels surround the intestines, but it makes sense when you realize that these blood vessels are how we get our nutrients into our bodies. Once absorbed into the bloodstream, our proteins, fats, carbohydrates, and vitamins can travel throughout the body via the blood vessels to be delivered wherever they are needed. The rest of the food and large amounts of liquid then travel to the large intestine (or colon), where water and small molecules called electrolytes can be absorbed. Then the remainder is eliminated (I'm assuming you're already familiar with this part). All of this movement through our digestive organs does not occur on its own or simply through gravity. The gastrointestinal tract depends on a series of coordinated muscle movements working in tandem to move nutrition through at a proper pace.

Our digestive system also depends heavily on a healthy gut microbiome, the bacteria that live in our digestive tract, primarily in the large intestine. Helpful bacteria in the colon help with the absorption of some nutrients as well as the production and absorption of certain vitamins. These good bacteria also help to prevent the growth of harmful bacteria in the gut. A robust concentration of gut bacteria, and the balance of the right *kind* of bacteria, is incredibly important for maintaining a healthy immune system as well as for effective and comfortable digestion. And, yes, the microbiome has even been shown to have an impact on our ability to lose and maintain a healthy weight.

This microbiome is influenced by the foods we eat, such as probiotics and prebiotics. Some foods, like high-quality yogurt and kimchi, contain live cultures of helpful bacteria. These are considered *pro*biotics. Other foods that contain nutrients such as fiber give the bacteria something to live on. These foods, like fresh fruits and vegetables, are considered *pre*biotics. It seems obvious how our nutrition can and does impact our gut biome, but perhaps surprisingly, researchers have also found that the gut microbiome changes in response to exercise. Several studies have now found that the gut microbiome of participants taking part in cardiovascular exercise improved in less than two months, particularly for participants with obesity.[22] This means that the balance of "good" bacteria—which aid in vitamin absorption and comfortable digestion—increased, while the types of bacteria associated with gastrointestinal pain, bloating, diarrhea, constipation, and even weight gain decreased. So, while our diet does play an important role in balancing the bacteria in our gut, we can shift our gut health for the better by adding exercise to our routine, independent of diet!

At the end of some of these studies, the researchers continued to follow participants as they went back to being sedentary, and results showed that the gut flora had shifted back to pre-exercise levels, emphasizing that we need to stay consistent with our physical activity in order to maintain healthy changes in our gut flora. Follow-up analysis of several similar studies also found a correlation between exercise and healthy gut flora, as well as a reduction in diseases including inflammatory bowel disease (IBD), irritable bowel syndrome (IBS), diverticulosis, and even cancer of the colon in the participants who exercised.[23]

Of course, many of our bodies' functions (and dysfunctions) depend on more than one kind of balance, and digestion is no exception. In addition to a healthy gut microbiome, we need the right concentration of digestive enzymes, chemicals, and even neurotransmitters to keep things working well and to avoid both discomfort and disease. I mentioned earlier that serotonin plays a role in healthy digestion by stimulating the movement of the smooth muscles in the digestive tract and influencing appetite. Scientists and clinicians have long thought of serotonin as an important brain chemical, but we now know that the majority of serotonin is produced in the gut and circulates within the digestive system. Serotonin receptors along the digestive pathway control the muscle contractions

---

[22] Morita et al., "Brisk Walking Increases Intestinal Bacteroides," 868; Allen et al., "Exercise Alters Gut Microbiota Composition," 747–57.

[23] Mailing et al., "Exercise and the Gut Microbiome," 75–85.

necessary to move food through the esophagus, stomach, small intestine, and the colon. This movement, which we call peristalsis, is necessary for digestion, and in conditions where peristalsis is slowed down, people complain of pain, bloating, constipation, and nausea. In some conditions caused by uncoordinated peristalsis, the intestines can twist or loop around themselves, causing pain, blockage of the digestive tract, and even death in severe cases. We already know that exercise increases serotonin levels and that this greatly affects our mental health. But this serotonin boost also keeps the bowel movements regular, countering constipation.

Increased serotonin in the gastrointestinal system also helps to dilate (or expand) the blood vessels that feed the digestive organs, bringing them increased oxygen and nutrients and removing waste more effectively. Serotonin also stimulates the secretion of certain digestive enzymes, helping us to break down our food and absorb nutrients. We now also know that there is a complicated collection of nerve cells throughout the digestive tract and that serotonin in the lining of these organs can promote the regeneration and survival of these neurons.[24] Many of us think of neurons as sensory organs, and they do carry sensation such as pain, discomfort, and pleasure to the spinal cord and brain. But neurons are also the outgoing messengers that tell muscles to flex, contract, or relax. So, with a system as complex as digestion, which relies on muscle contractions in a specifically timed sequence, these muscle-driving neurons have an incredibly important job to do, one that we literally depend on for survival.

We talked earlier about the nervous system in terms of our fight-or-flight response, or sympathetic nervous system response, which makes us feel jittery and directs the body to increase heart rate and breathing as well as deprioritize digestion and growth. The opposite system, our parasympathetic nervous system, is often referred to as the rest-and-digest response. During exercise, we want to tap into the sympathetic nervous system response to help our bodies move more

---

[24] Mawe and Hoffman, "Serotonin Signalling in the Gut," 473–86.

effectively and maximize our strength and endurance. After exercise is over, the body, which always seeks balance, shifts into parasympathetic mode to rest and recover and stimulate digestion so that we can absorb the nutrients we need to fight-and-flight another day.

In my clinical practice, I see many patients with chronic constipation with or without IBS. They are in pain and desperate to regulate their digestive schedules. I have seen firsthand that exercise reduces episodes of constipation, and that lack of physical activity is associated with a higher incidence of constipation. Since we know now that our gut bacteria and our serotonin levels both play an important role in reducing constipation and gastrointestinal pain, this is no surprise.

Several studies have examined IBS symptoms as well as other measures of quality of life in patients who suffer with this condition. They have found that participants who exercised at least twenty to thirty minutes per day experienced far fewer symptoms of IBS, particularly constipation, and also reported improvements in overall quality of life.[25] This is good news for many of my patients who come in thinking that they have to take medication every day or at least several days a month in order to feel comfortable and experience regular bathroom habits.

I remember a particular young man that came to see me complaining of IBS and constipation symptoms. He was clearly frustrated and uncomfortable. This young man, let's call him Alex, was resigned to the idea that he may have to start on medications and that this would likely be a lifelong routine for him. After discussing some lifestyle factors, I discovered that Alex worked in food service, so he was on his feet often, but he did not engage in any routine exercise. He was busy trying to finish college, so he felt that he did not have much free time for physical activity or meal prep. He frequently ate at the restaurant where he worked or would grab fast food on his way between work and classes. We talked for a while and discussed

---

[25] Fani et al., "The Effect of Aerobic Exercises," 161–5; Johannesson et al., "Intervention to Increase Physical Activity," 600–8.

the fact that, yes, there are pills that many people with his symptoms can take to help relieve the symptoms of bloating, stomach cramps, and constipation. But he would have to take the medication every day, possibly for the rest of his life, to maintain relief from these symptoms. As an alternative, I recommended that we start a one-month trial of diet changes and brisk twenty- to thirty-minute walks at least four days a week.

Thanks to diligent effort on his part (and motivation to avoid starting on daily pills at his young age), Alex was able to make these changes, and he reported back one month later that he felt so much better. He was no longer experiencing constant bloating or painful constipation. He also stated that he had more energy even though he still stayed up late studying for his classes on occasion. We still get to check in from time to time, and Alex has told me on a couple of occasions that he had fallen into bad habits once or twice since then, but he feels the difference in his symptoms and knows that it means it's time to get himself back up and start on his regular exercise and nutrition again. He knows he will feel better! If you already suffer from IBS and/or constipation, I know that taking a walk is the last thing you feel like doing during an episode of stomach cramps, but I promise that you will feel better once you do.

Speaking of painful gastrointestinal conditions, another one of the most painful yet common GI conditions I see in my practice is gallstones with inflammation of the gallbladder. Exercise helps move bile through the digestive tract and thus prevent the formation of gallstones, which can be not only painful, but also cause inflammation of the gallbladder, bile ducts, and the pancreas, known as pancreatitis. In addition, exercise decreases our bad cholesterols such as LDL and triglycerides and raises our good cholesterol or HDL. Since the majority of gallstones in Western countries are made of cholesterol crystals, it makes sense that lowering our cholesterol levels would decrease our likelihood of developing gallstones. We also see a decrease in gallstone formation in patients who have higher

HDL. Less exercise equals lower HDL, which in turn equals a higher chance of forming gallstones.[26] As anyone who has experienced gallstones or pancreatitis would tell you, any means to prevent such a painful condition is well worth it!

It may seem like digestion is one small bodily function among many. However, I find that it is impossible to overstate the extent to which digestion affects our overall sense of well-being. Perhaps this has to do with the communication between the gut and the brain in the so-called gut-brain axis, or it may simply be due to the fact that when digestion is working properly, we absorb nutrients and remove waste at the proper rate for the rest of our bodily functions. Conversely, when digestion is not working properly, my patients complain not only of diarrhea, constipation, nausea, or heartburn, but they also feel physical pain in the rest of the body as well as an overall sense of malaise. This means the body is not removing waste or absorbing nutrients effectively. So, their entire body feels out of whack.

Movement keeps this system in balance by optimizing our serotonin levels as well as allowing the autonomic nervous system to shift properly between fight or flight and rest and digest. We need to move in order for these systems to function properly and to feel good!

---

[26] Shanmugam et al., "Modulating Lipid Metabolism," 99–110.

CHAPTER 6

Memory

I hear a lot of my patients, even very young patients, complain about lapses in memory and focus, forgetting names or words frequently. Some of these lapses are clear signs of stress but also of less-than-ideal lifestyle factors that affect our cognition. Lack of sleep, poor nutrition, and constant multitasking all affect our mental sharpness, and we could easily write an entirely separate book about the lifestyle factors that affect our memory. For now, we will continue our focus on how physical activity comes into play. The good news is that fitting in some time for exercise ultimately improves our memory, both in the short and long term. This fact alone kept me consistent with getting outside or on a treadmill regularly during those long days of lectures and study sessions for PA school.

Studies have demonstrated that people who were given lists to memorize and participated in mild to moderate cardiovascular exercise did better recalling their lists versus their counterparts who were given the same lists and then given the opportunity to just sit and relax before or after studying. One of these studies was conducted recently by David Marchant and colleagues at Edge Hill University and Manchester University.[27] In Marchant's study, healthy adults were divided into quiet rest or moderate-intensity exercise groups before they were

---

[27] Marchant et al., "Acute Moderate and High Intensity Exercise," 1716.

given a task to memorize. The group that exercised outperformed the sedentary group in accurately recalling their lists of material. So we actually remember new information better if we jog or bike or swim as opposed to sitting still before learning something.

As memory is still quite difficult to understand, we're not sure why this is. It may have something to do with the diminishing stress hormones like cortisol and adrenaline, or an increase in beneficial substances such as neuropeptide Y. Remember that neuropeptide Y is found in high concentrations in the hippocampus, which happens to be the area of the brain that plays the largest role in our memory. Perhaps the increase in blood flow to the brain as our circulation speeds up makes the entire organ function better. Whatever the reason, the effect of exercise on improving memory is measurable. I used this to my advantage many times in PA school before a difficult test or an anticipated heavy or long lecture class. After so many minutes or hours of studying, I knew that I could not absorb much more new material anyway, and it not only felt great to get up and move, but it actually helped me remember what I had just studied and absorb the next set of material more accurately.

Perhaps even more profoundly, exercise has been shown to help with memory over time, including reducing the chances of developing dementia. One factor in this may be that the size of the hippocampus (the primary area of the brain associated with memory) actually increases with physical activity. In normal aging, the size of the brain reduces slowly over time. But in recent studies, people who were advised to exercise and were monitored over the course of a year actually showed a 2 percent *increase* in the size of the hippocampus, in short reversing about two years of normal age-related decline.[28] It seems incredible that physical activity could help an organ like the brain to literally age in reverse, but that is exactly what happens!

Several other studies done over the last ten to fifteen years have noted an increasing importance in lifestyle factors, particularly

---

[28] Erickson et al., "Exercise Training Increases Size of Hippocampus," 3017-22.

exercise, in preventing what was previously thought to be expected age-related decline in memory, including the widely publicized FINGER study (the Finnish Geriatric Intervention Study to Prevent Cognitive Impairment and Disability).[29] One of the most popular studies on memory of our time, the FINGER study was based on the neuropsychiatric battery of tests and conducted over a two-year period in 2009–2011. The 1,200 participants in the experimental group engaged in progressively frequent aerobic exercise that was tailored to their preferences and included activities like jogging, Nordic walking, aqua gym, or gymnastics, eventually building up to five to six times a week. They also engaged in strength training exercises at the gym, guided by physiotherapists for the first six months. The participants in this group showed greater improvements in their cognitive test scores compared to their peers in the control group who were given only standard medical advice over the same period of time.

I remember my grandmother faithfully completing crossword puzzles on a daily basis to help keep her mind and memory sharp. I wish I could have told her then that a thirty-minute walk or a trip to the gym would have been even more beneficial.

Another analysis of several studies found that exercise, especially if started in middle age, could reduce the incidence of dementia by as much as 30 percent, and as much as 45 percent for Alzheimer's disease in particular.[30] In this analysis, a study done in Wales over a period of thirty-five years, exercise was the most powerful factor in reducing dementia even when compared to other healthy lifestyle modifications such as a healthy diet, moderate alcohol intake, avoidance of smoking, and maintaining healthy body weight.[31] Of course, adding at least four out of five of these other factors had an even greater preventative impact. But I cannot stress enough that

---

[29] Kivipelto et al., "The Finnish Geriatric Intervention Study," 657–65.
[30] Iso-Markku et al., "Physical Activity As a Protective Factor," 701–9.
[31] Elwood, et al., "Chronic Diseases and Dementia."

even when measured separately from healthy body weight, regular exercise carried the single biggest influence on reducing the chances of developing dementia. Yet again, the scale is not the most important factor—exercise is! And the benefits are better and better the sooner we start and the more consistent we remain.

It is also never too late to start exercising to reap some benefit. The Alzheimer's Society particularly stresses the importance of exercise later in life, and reports that for people in their eighties, the least active 10 percent of people were more than twice as likely to suffer from Alzheimer's disease compared to the most active 10 percent.[32]

While preventing dementia or cognitive decline later in life is a long-term benefit, and we are mostly concerned with the immediate results, I mention this because dementia is quickly becoming one of the most frustrating disease states to encounter. Many of us will be affected by dementia, either personally or as the friend or relative of someone dealing with it, and to date, there is no cure and little treatment to even slow the progression. It is one of the most horrible diseases to face, as the slow decline disrupts our activities, our relationships, and our livelihoods. So many of my patients who have supported a friend or relative through a dementia diagnosis come in asking what they can do to avoid it, and among the risk factors that we can control, getting regular physical activity is the most beneficial. And again, our physical activity also helps with our memory in the short term as well. Our brains literally function better on the days that we exercise and will continue to function better in the years to come. This is another reason I get up early to get a good workout in before the day starts. I feel that I owe it to my patients to be as mentally sharp as possible!

---

[32] Alzheimer's Society, "Physical Activity and the Risk of Dementia."

ACETYLCHOLINE

Earlier we discussed several chemicals that affect our body, brain function, and particularly our mood. I want to mention another neurotransmitter called acetylcholine, which plays a significant role in our memory. Acetylcholine is essential for focused attention and the encoding of new information. It facilitates communication between neurons (brain cells), which is critical for learning new tasks and consolidating information. Acetylcholine is also involved in the process of transferring information from short-term to long-term memory. This consolidation is crucial for retaining new information over time. Since attention is critical for encoding information into memory, disruptions in acetylcholine signaling can impact how well we remember things.

One of the hallmark features of Alzheimer's disease is a significant decrease in acetylcholine levels. This reduction correlates with the memory loss and cognitive decline characteristic of the disease. Medications used to treat Alzheimer's often aim to increase acetylcholine levels or mimic its action to help manage symptoms.

In the context of physical exercise, acetylcholine is crucial for muscle contraction. It is released from the endings of nerves that control muscle movement and binds to receptors on muscle cells, leading to muscle contraction. Efficient release and reception of acetylcholine is essential for smooth, coordinated movements, so it's logical that regular exercise is known to boost acetylcholine levels in the body and, in turn, the brain. This increase in acetylcholine enhances cognitive functions such as memory, attention, and learning. Studies suggest that physical exercise, especially aerobic activities like running or cycling, can increase the density of acetylcholine receptors in the brain and improve overall brain health.[33] This likely contributes to the cognitive benefits associated with regular physical activity, such as improved memory.

---

[33] Zong et al., "Physical Exercise Improves Alzheimer›s Disease," 869507.

Of course, memory is a complicated thing, and there are so many factors that go into our ability to remember clearly and accurately. Our sleep, emotional health, the size of the hippocampus and prefrontal cortex, and the right balance of neurotransmitter chemicals in the brain all play a role.

We know that exercise helps to regulate our emotions and facilitates improved sleep. We know that exercise increases the size of the hippocampus, countering the normal aging process, which shrinks the hippocampus over time. And we see a reduction in stress chemicals and an increase in beneficial neurochemicals. Just as with our emotional regulation, there are several factors at work, and no single factor can claim more importance than others. However, we do know that one thing positively influences all of them: exercise!

CHAPTER 7

What About Pain?

One of the reasons that many people avoid exercise is fear of pain. But for those who already suffer from chronic pain and are concerned about it worsening, there is great news! Studies show that over the long term, a regular exercise routine will actually reduce pain in the body.

Several clinical trials have shown that exercise effectively reduces pain from a variety of chronic conditions, including fibromyalgia, osteoarthritis ("wear-and-tear arthritis"), myofascial syndromes, low-back pain, chronic fatigue syndrome, and even dysmenorrhea (painful periods). There are several reasons why this is true, some of them having to do with the condition of the muscles and balance of muscle tone in the body, some of them having to do with the body's chemistry changes in response to exercise, and some of them having to do with changes to receptors in the nerves and brain itself.

Most impressively, many of the participants in these studies already suffered from some form of chronic pain prior to taking part in the study. Several of those participants were interviewed before the trials began and were skeptical that they would even be able to complete the physical activity being asked of them. But at the end of the studies, they were delighted to report not only reduced pain but also a life-changing sense of freedom that came with movement.

One of my patients, let's call her Martha, entered into her own exercise program with similar skepticism. She had become used to a certain amount of pain due to a combination of rheumatoid arthritis and spinal stenosis that had left her joints achy and swollen. She used a walker for any excursions out of the house so she could lean on something to relieve her back pain after too many steps. She also took a combination of narcotic and anti-inflammatory pain medications as well as muscle relaxers, nerve pain blockers, biologic antirheumatic medication, and sleep medications at night. Her daytime routine became increasingly sedentary due to her pain. At one point during some routine screening, we discovered that Martha's bone density had declined into a condition called osteoporosis, which placed her at a much higher risk of breaking a bone, particularly in the hips, wrist, or spine. What I did not realize at that time was that Martha's sister had suffered a hip fracture two years earlier and had eventually died due to complications from that fracture. Martha was determined to do everything she could to improve her bone density, decrease her fracture risk, and avoid the painful decline she witnessed in her sister.

We discussed weight-bearing exercise, and at first, as I mentioned earlier, she was skeptical that she would be able to manage any exercise at all, but she was motivated. Working with her other specialists, we decided on a course of physical therapy that would involve a combination of core strengthening for her abdominal and back muscles, treadmill walking, and full-body resistance training. We set a goal of thirty minutes of exercise three to four days per week, which at first was quite difficult for her. Amazingly, after six months of this program, she reported that she was now walking on the treadmill at a steep incline (further increasing her leg strength and bone density) and that she was no longer needing her walker at all. Even more amazingly, she had been able to stop all of her narcotic pain medications and sleep medications, as well as wean herself off her other medications for pain. She stated that at first this was intentional because she didn't want to feel too sleepy during her exercise sessions, but she found that over time she did not need them as frequently. I remember this day with her for many reasons, but mostly for the look on her face when she told me that, six months prior, she thought I was absolutely crazy for thinking she could ever walk for thirty minutes! And now she was doing that and then some several times a week and feeling great doing it.

MECHANICAL

Many of my patients, like Martha at first, seem to believe that exercise will lead to lasting pain or injury. I often hear things like "I can't run because it will hurt my knees" or "I'm afraid that I will hurt my old shoulder injury if I lift weights." Sure, some temporary strain or soreness is common with exercise, especially when first starting out or changing up your routine or intensity level. But over the long term, exercise will have the opposite effect, actually reducing pain.

A systematic review of over fifty clinical trials found that people who exercise regularly actually reduce their risk of joint pain from arthritis over time.[34] The review focused mostly on osteoarthritis of the knees and found high-quality evidence in forty-four randomized controlled trials that the exercise groups reported far less knee pain from arthritis both during the period of exercise intervention and for between two to six months afterward.

Over my years of clinical practice, I have observed that, at a mechanical level, one large source of pain is imbalance surrounding the joints and skeletal structures in our bodies. Our muscles allow movement by pulling the skeleton in different directions around an articulation or joint. In a perfect scenario, there should be a balance of muscle tone on each of the opposing sides of the body so that the

---

[34] Fransen et al., "Exercise for Osteoarthritis of the Knee," 1554–7.

skeleton is completely relaxed at rest with no overriding tension on either side of the bones or joints. But often a particular muscle or muscle group will shorten, either from overuse or lack of countering force from the opposite side, and this will pull the skeleton out of alignment. This leads to chronic joint pain, especially in areas like the knees and shoulders, and even around the back, neck, and hips. For example, the iliopsoas, a deep hip-flexor muscle that runs from the lower back and top of the pelvic bone to the front of the thigh, is contracted, or shortened, when we sit, and many of us sit for long periods of time. Without regular breaks to stretch or lengthen out, and without proper support from the other abdominal and lower-back muscles or counterbalance from the core muscles, the iliopsoas becomes shortened and tight, making it painful to stand or fully stretch the hip joint after a prolonged period of sitting. This creates chronic lower-back, hip, and groin pain.

Muscle imbalance also commonly creates pain in the front of the shoulder after years of rolling the shoulders forward into the chest as we carry things in front of the body, reach forward to grasp objects, or simply let our posture slump. The pectoral muscles in the top of the chest and front of the shoulder become shortened and pull the shoulder forward while the lower trapezius muscles and rhomboids in the mid-upper back that should be pulling the shoulder back and down become overstretched and weakened, eventually failing to offer countersupport to the shoulder.

A proper exercise routine can help to reverse this mechanical pain both by strengthening the opposing or balancing muscle groups and stretching or lengthening the areas prone to shortening. It may be worthwhile to meet with a trainer or physical therapist, or take a class under the eyes of a trained instructor who can watch for proper technique and help you spot a muscle imbalance. The good news for most of us with limited time or resources is that a one-on-one trainer isn't required to achieve muscle-balancing benefits. Participants in the studies mentioned earlier were generally instructed to exercise, and even in cases where they were monitored closely during exercise sessions, they were not given individual or specific technique instruction. Yet they still achieved a decrease in their pain.

I often walk through some simple stretches and exercises with my patients who come in complaining of joint or muscle pain, and many are able to follow through with this routine at home. For others who need more hands-on guidance, physical therapy is a great place to start. A well-trained therapist may employ some manual techniques to facilitate the healing process, break up muscle adhesions, and the like, but they will also walk through a series of stretching and strengthening exercises aimed at balancing the body and supporting the joints.

Movement also stimulates our joints to create something called synovial fluid, which functions essentially like a lubricant. I sometimes refer to this as nature's version of the Tin Man's oil can. Synovial fluid is a rich, viscous fluid full of proteins that reduces friction in between the bones and absorbs some of the impact of movement, allowing the joints to move smoothly. It also brings nutrients such as hyaluronic acid and lubricin into the joint, keeping the cartilage and joints healthy. As we move, the mechanical force on the joint capsule stimulates the synovial membrane to produce more of this fluid, and with regular movement, the entire joint capsule receives the nutrients it needs to function optimally.

Exercise also increases blood flow to working muscles, which helps deliver nutrients and remove wastes and toxins. When we exercise, our muscle cells use energy in the form of ATP molecules. As we use this energy, our body creates waste products, namely carbon dioxide (CO_2) and sometimes lactic acid. Because CO_2 causes blood vessels to dilate, the body has an amazing ability to increase blood flow to the areas that need it most. This allows the circulatory system to gather up more waste and carry it back to the lungs where we exhale it out or to the kidneys where we expel it in urine. The increased blood flow also brings more oxygen and other nutrients to the working muscles so they can continue to work and repair. This is one of the reasons that active recovery, or cool down (continued mild- to moderate-paced exercise), actually helps reduce muscle soreness that comes from strenuous or intense exercise. Moderate exercise also helps to flush out the toxins built up in our tight muscles from prolonged sitting or clenching. Think of how good it feels to stand up and move your legs and core after you have been cramped up in a car for several hours on a road trip. Our muscles need blood flow, and they need to move to get enough of it!

It is important to note that most of the data showing decreased pain in response to exercise is focused on *chronic* pain, so we need to make a distinction between the chronic-pain conditions discussed above and acute pain. By chronic pain, I am referring to long-lasting pain that may involve most of the body or any single area as in the muscle-imbalance scenario. It may be noticeable as a number of different sensations such as dull or achy, but it is rarely sharp or shooting. It can be constant or peak and subside with certain activities or positions, but in general, chronic pain means pain that occurs daily or nearly every day for over a few weeks at a time.

Acute pain, meaning a sudden onset of new pain that involves a particular area, may indicate an injury, and this needs a different kind of attention. If you notice a new type of pain that occurs repeatedly with the same type of movement, please seek medical attention to have it evaluated further. In some cases acute pain can indicate a simple strain or sprain and may heal easily with time and proper stretching, but it can also indicate a skeletal issue such as malalignment or an injury such as a stress fracture. Depending on the severity, such injuries may require a period of rest along with some compression, ice, and anti-inflammatory meds. Some types of these injuries, sprains for example, actually heal faster with continued gentle range of motion rather than complete rest. We used to recommend that patients completely rest every type of injury, but we know now that this is wrong! Studies actually show us that continued movement is important for several types of injuries to heal more quickly and with less pain along the way. Moving through mild to moderate pain increases the blood flow to the injured areas, bringing nutrients to the injury that allow it to heal, and it also increases the right kinds of chemicals that the body needs for repair, including testosterone, which we discussed earlier. Movement also allows the surrounding tissues to maintain a proper balance of strength and flexibility so that the injured area is supported rather than "frozen" or in a state where it becomes increasingly tight and inflexible. This is one of the many reasons that medical practitioners have shifted away from advising patients to immobilize every injury and rather to move gently and constantly to allow for better healing.

Of course, exercise can also help prevent these types of acute injury from occurring in the first place. As mentioned earlier, proper exercise technique can help to stabilize the body by building equal strength on either side of the bones and joints so that the skeleton is better able to handle stress and movement. For example, having a routine that includes both calf and tibialis (the muscle that runs along the shin) strengthening can help to stabilize the ankles, so that a simple trip and fall that may have caused an ankle sprain in normal conditions may only cause a temporary loss of balance. This happened to me once several years ago as I used to be very prone to twisting my right ankle. But a year later after training for a mud run with some friends, I stepped in yet another pothole (yes, I am fairly accident-prone). However, this time I did not injure the ankle; I merely wobbled for a moment and was able to go on running. The support muscles that I had built up around the lower leg were able to counter the stress applied to the outside of the ankle and hold it in position with minimal bend. I was so thankful for all those repeated calf raises and toe taps that day!

Balance and core-stabilization exercises are also extremely helpful for preventing injury to the spine as well as preventing falls. Core strength involves the abdominal muscles (the coveted six-pack abs) as well as the sides of the waist, lower back, gluteal muscles, and thighs. Exercises such as Pilates and yoga are wonderful for targeting these areas. I have recently become a huge fan of Pilates classes in particular. One reason is that I leave every class feeling accomplished and strong but also stretched out, as if I had just gotten a massage and a workout all in one. Even more importantly, the core muscles that Pilates develops have improved my speed and strength in other sports while preventing injury. So naturally, I encourage my patients, especially those who report twinges of back pain, hip pain, or knee pain with walking or exercising, to add Pilates to their routine. Even movements such as walking can help to strengthen the core, especially if you walk with your torso properly lifted by your abdominal and back muscles. A strong core can even help prevent injury to the arms and legs by supporting the hips and shoulder girdle so the extremities are not tasked with stabilizing the body while working. This helps to make strength gains in the arms and legs easier over time, and movement actually begins to feel easier and more comfortable throughout the body.

Core strength also helps us to recover from falls and injuries more easily. One of my favorite examples of this is a patient whom I have known for years. We'll call him Robert. Robert's story actually exemplifies several key points of this book. When I met him, he was an older gentleman with a few medical conditions, including high blood pressure and heart disease, but he came in to see me for the first time after pulling a muscle in his lower back from, of all things, falling backward while leaning over to whisper something sweet to his wife. Robert recovered gradually, with the help of physical therapy and some treatments for pain, but he used a cane off and on after that point, and the pain would act up from time to time.

Over the next few years, life was not kind to Robert. A cancer diagnosis and a sudden, rapid decline in his wife's health hit him extremely hard. He seemed depressed, understandably so, and he relied more and more on his cane.

One day during a visit, he mentioned a new health center opening up near his home, and he told me that after his appointment, he was planning to head over there and sign up for a membership. I thought this was a great idea and encouraged him to follow through with it. We discussed the fact that both the exercise and the social interaction would be great for his mood, and it has been! He did sign up, and he decided to ride the stationary bike and follow a weight-training circuit, at first twice and then three times a week. He found that he really enjoyed it and that it gave him something to look forward to, especially on days when he visited his wife, who was now in long-term care with rapidly declining memory. Some of those visits were particularly disheartening, so his gym sessions became a nice stress relief.

He seemed more cheerful over the next couple of months to be sure. And impressively, he began to come in for his appointments without his cane. His posture and walking gait both looked more fluid, more comfortable. He told me with a somewhat coy smile during one of our visits that he had fallen recently, for the first time in a while. But his smile widened as he went on to say: "And you know what? I got right up off the floor without any help, and it wasn't even difficult. I don't think I could have done that a few months ago." Those repetitions had strengthened his muscles, especially his core, enough to support his previously injured back in daily movement but also to recover from a fall that in the past would have left him vulnerable on the floor. I believe he was absolutely right!

CHEMICAL

We have already discussed the power of endorphins and enkephalins in decreasing emotional distress, but these chemicals also bind to physical pain-killing receptors in our bodies as well. The term endorphins actually applies to about twenty different peptide hormones, which are primarily produced in the pituitary gland. When we exercise, the brain and body perceive that stress is occurring, and another part of the brain, the hypothalamus, which essentially acts as the pituitary gland's boss, releases corticotropin-releasing hormone, or CRH. CRH signals the pituitary gland to start making corticotropin, otherwise known as adrenocorticotropic hormone (ACTH), as well as proteins that will become endorphins and enkephalins. These endorphins and enkephalins then bind to opioid receptors (off buttons for pain in the nervous system). In the peripheral nervous system (nerves connected to the muscles of the body), endorphins also help to decrease pain by lowering pain-increasing proteins such as substance P. They also bind to receptors in the central nervous system (the brain) that increase dopamine, the neurotransmitter associated with desire and motivation. Again, we have discussed how these chemicals affect us emotionally, but these chemicals also play an important role in how we experience physical pain. When we move, our bodies respond by releasing chemicals that we need in order to help movement feel more comfortable, to help our body feel good.

On the contrary, inactivity essentially lowers the pain threshold by having the opposite effect on pain-regulating chemicals and receptors in our bodies.[35] Sedentary lifestyles are associated with lower levels of endorphins and the building-block proteins that make them, as well as decreased availability of opioid receptors that receive the endorphin signals. Our bodies are amazingly efficient and good at learning what might be needed at any given moment. So, if we routinely tap into a certain system, the body responds by keeping it primed and ready to go. But if our bodies perceive that a certain system is not often used, we will conserve energy by underutilizing that process, which in the case of a sedentary lifestyle means having fewer endorphin-precursor proteins and opioid receptors primed and ready for use.

We have also already mentioned that exercise lowers chronic cortisol levels, or stress-hormone levels, and discussed how cortisol affects mental health as well as physical health. Studies have also shown that elevated cortisol levels lead to lower pain tolerance.[36]

---

[35] Hanna et al., "Impact of Sedentary Behavior," 1265814.
[36] Trevino et al., "Decreased Cortisol and Development of Chronic Pain," 286–92.

This is somewhat ironic since, initially, cortisol acts as an *anti-*inflammatory in the body. Many theorize that after the initial phase, if cortisol levels remain elevated, this hormone will stop binding to its main target receptor, GR (or glucocorticoid receptor), and will be increasingly attracted to the mineralocorticoid receptor (MR), which has *pro-*inflammatory effects. Another widely accepted theory, the glucocorticoid resistance model, suggests that continuously elevated levels of cortisol can reduce the sensitivity of certain cells to its anti-inflammatory effects. This results in persistent inflammation despite the presence of cortisol.[37]

Another chemical involved in increased pain is prostaglandin. Prostaglandins are fatty acids that function like hormones in the body, that is, they facilitate a reaction. In normal circumstances, prostaglandins are required for repair of damaged tissue, formation of blood clots, bringing on labor, and a number of other necessary bodily functions. However, in high levels, prostaglandins cause increased pain (think of labor pains or even painful menstrual cramps as an example). Not surprisingly, the body's stress response triggers an increase in prostaglandins. If there is a true threat approaching, we would need these prostaglandins to protect and repair any tissues that might be damaged in the act of fighting or fleeing from danger. But with chronic stress increasing these pain-inducing chemicals, we are not reaping any benefit, only feeling the pain. Prostaglandins on their own have a short half-life, so they will dissipate over a short period of time, but as any woman who suffers from painful menstrual cycles can attest, the pain can keep returning in waves so that it feels constant! Thankfully, the beta endorphins produced during exercise can also help to wash out these prostaglandins. In fact, studies have shown that a consistent routine of moderate cardiovascular activity helps to reduce the severity of menstrual cramps,[38] and this is likely due to the decrease in prostaglandins.

---

[37] Malesu, "Cortisol, Inflammation, and Disease."
[38] Dehnavi et al., "Effect of Aerobic Exercise on Primary Dysmenorrhea," 3.

A large body of evidence links increased emotional stress with increased physical pain. Although the exact reasons are difficult to pinpoint, it seems to involve a combination of the factors discussed here, including the balance of chemicals like prostaglandin, cortisol, and endorphins. The fact that pain itself is also a stressor creates a vicious cycle of pain and emotional distress that is hard to break, especially if one stuck in this cycle is convinced that movement makes the pain worse. By getting up and getting moving, we can begin to reverse this cycle. We literally just need to take the first step!

I met a woman recently who, after several emergency room visits for various aches and pains, had been given everything from anti-inflammatory medicines to muscle relaxers to steroids and topical numbing treatments. She was, by then, also taking more than one narcotic pain medication. Her granddaughter, who brought her to the office visit, expressed that she could not understand why her grandmother was still in pain since she was completely sedentary and therefore very unlikely to injure anything. And it was true—in all of the emergency room visits and X-rays and CT scans that had been done, no major injury was ever identified aside from some mild arthritis. The women both told me that they assumed rest was good for the body, so this patient thought she should move as little as possible all day long. It was quite an alarming thing for me to hear—of course she was in pain! Yes, she had some mild arthritis from living into her seventh decade of life, but her answer to anything that hurt was to sit completely still, and as far as I could tell, she had been doing this for several years.

Without movement, her body lacked healthy blood flow, which brings oxygen and nutrients to the muscles, joints, and other connective tissues, as well as carries away waste. It was amazing that she had not developed a blood clot! She had also been living with higher levels of every pro-inflammatory chemical the body could produce and lacking every natural pain-killing response to balance it. So instead, she relied on medications, and still she felt pain despite taking them regularly.

We need rest, yes, but we need periods of movement before this rest in order for our bodies to function optimally.

NEUROLOGIC

Pain, like all sensory input, is carried in signals from sensory nerves to particular areas in the brain. It seems like a simple one-way street. If you prick your finger, the sharp sensation goes straight up that nerve from the fingertip to the spinal cord and into the sensory cortex of the brain. But it's not quite that simple. The incoming signals also have to pass through the brain stem, which acts as a gatekeeper for information in and out of the brain and inhibits (or silences) certain signals. A particular area of the brain stem known as the rostral ventromedial medulla (RVM) plays a major role in relaying sensory information from the body to the sensory cortex of the brain and is thought to be the key to either increased or decreased pain perception.[39] In response to exercise, this area of the brain stem actually increases the presence of certain receptors including opioid, serotonin, and cannabinoid receptors,[40] meaning that this area of the brain is creating new places for pain-killing chemicals to land, effectively opening our bodies up for a dose of natural pain relief (without the negative side effects of medicinal painkillers).

Some chronic-pain conditions, such as fibromyalgia, are thought to be caused by hyperactive sensory nerves, meaning that they send the brain messages of pain more often than normal, and sometimes with no obvious underlying cause. We are still not sure what causes this, but we do know that exercise is the single best treatment for patients with fibromyalgia.

I had a patient once who did not start having fibromyalgia

---

[39] Pagliusi Jr. et al., "Rostral Ventromedial Medulla in Stress Responses," 776.
[40] Lima et al., "Does Exercise Increase or Decrease Pain?" 4141–50.

symptoms until she became sedentary. She noticed that she was feeling pain all over her body and set herself up with a rheumatologist thinking that she must have developed either rheumatoid arthritis, lupus, or some other similar condition that was spreading pain and inflammation all over her body. The rheumatologist did a thorough workup, and when everything came back negative, he informed her that she actually had fibromyalgia. He offered several medications including antidepressants and muscle relaxers, but she did not want to start any of these, fearing the side effects and not thrilled about needing medications to avoid pain on a daily basis.

We talked as I reviewed the workup that the specialist had done, and one key point in her story came up. Her symptoms started earlier that year when some construction began on the grounds of the school where she worked as a teacher. This meant that she couldn't go out for her customary twenty-minute walk at lunchtime that had been part of her routine for twenty-plus years. By the time the construction ended, she was out of the habit of going on this daily walk, and the Texas heat seemed particularly oppressive that year, so she had not resumed the routine. Her nervous system was now missing the stimulation from her walks and was therefore firing off random signals throughout her body, making everything hurt. She had no other input to act on the rest of the sensory system and very little to stimulate the movement neurons, so her brain and body were left concentrating on nothing but unpleasant sensations, and her brain stem, which had previously been full of naturally pain-killing compounds and receptors, had let these helpful pieces atrophy. No wonder she felt that everything hurt! I could see the light bulb moment on her entire face when she came to the realization that the interruption in her walking routine coincided with the start of her pain symptoms. She agreed to try resuming the midday walks and to follow up with me in a month to see if her pain levels improved.

As you might guess, in a month she was feeling quite a bit better, and she was able to stay off medication. She told me at her follow-up appointment that she hadn't realized before that she was accustomed to small aches and pains now and then, but she had learned to tolerate them. Without her walks, she felt more frequent and more intense pains that made every little annoyance so much more aggravating. Now that she was back on her walking routine, her pain was decreased to a tolerable level that she could manage with just the occasional over-the-counter anti-inflammatory, no strong or sedating daily medications needed.

Several studies demonstrate similar results to those that my patient experienced. In fact, one meta-analysis in the journal *Scientific Reports* looked at eighteen studies published on fibromyalgia symptoms and exercise and found that several forms of exercise, including aerobic exercise, resistance training, and flexibility or stretching exercises all helped to alleviate pain and improve quality of life for patients with fibromyalgia.[41] Aerobic exercise in particular decreased pain levels as well as depression in the study subjects, but any form of movement, including stretching and strength training, improved the participants' physical quality of life.

So, we can see that exercise at a mechanical level can help with pain by increasing blood flow, circulating nutrients, and building balanced muscle tone. At a chemical level, exercise can help control pain signals by increasing the feel-good chemicals and decreasing the noxious ones. Exercise also helps to regulate how we receive signals from our nervous system. This helps to control pain found in conditions from arthritis to irritable bowel syndrome, from menstrual cramps to fibromyalgia.

So yes, "motion is lotion," to borrow the trending phrase. It is also armor building, joint protecting, nervous-system regulating, and pain-chemical killing. In short, exercise is the best treatment we have for our chronic aches and pains. We may experience some temporary strain, soreness, and fatigue, but ultimately, moving our bodies more will promote long-lasting relief from chronic pain!

---

[41] Couto et al., "Effect of Different Types of Exercise," 10391.

CHAPTER 8

Getting Going

Whether you are just starting out, have been exercising for a while, or are trying to ramp up your fitness routine, there are some benchmarks that experts tell us we should be shooting for. Medical professionals and fitness experts generally recommend 150 minutes a week of cardiovascular exercise for heart health, which breaks down to thirty minutes five days per week. By cardiovascular exercise, I mean any activity that gets the heart rate up to 60–80 percent of your maximum heart rate. You can estimate your maximum heart rate by subtracting your age from 220. So, a twenty-year-old's maximum heart rate would be 200. A sixty-year-old's maximum heart rate would be 160. That would mean that an ideal cardiovascular exercise heart rate for the said sixty-year-old would be 60–80 percent of 160, or 96–128 beats per minute. For the twenty-year-old with a maximum heart rate of 200, a cardio training zone would fall between 120–160 beats per minute. Of course, this is a rough estimate, and not all twenty-somethings or sixty-somethings are at the same level of fitness to begin with.

Another way to judge whether you are in the cardio fitness zone is by your perceived exertion. In general, at a mild to moderate exertion, you should be able to hold a conversation but may start to feel a little winded while speaking. This will tell you that you're working hard enough to reap the benefits of cardiovascular exercise, but not so hard that it would be impossible to continue for thirty minutes. At high-intensity exercise, you should be too short of breath to hold a conversation. At this level, you would likely be working at a heart rate approaching your maximum, and it is usually only sustainable for a few minutes at a time, depending on your fitness level. A more precise estimate of your current maximum heart rate can be obtained by seeing your doctor for a VO_2 max test or exercise stress test. This test can also give you a good idea of your current fitness level and let you know how much room there is for improvement.

We know there are massive physical health benefits noted when we exercise at a moderate intensity for roughly thirty minutes, five days per week, but even shorter or fewer sessions can have a major impact and get you started toward feeling better in your body. It makes me laugh that the cardiology studies I have read in school and in the years since graduating generally all used a gold standard of 150 minutes of exercise per week, while many of the neurology studies I came across asked only 120 minutes of exercise per week of their participants. (Are the neurologists and cardiologists secretly at war with one another?) The important takeaway for all of us is that those studies with a shorter duration or fewer days still showed benefits.

You should measure your success by how your body feels, by how deeply you sleep at night, and by how calm you feel throughout the day. Can you move comfortably? Can you get up and down from a low chair or from the floor with minimal effort?

There is no one-size-fits-all treatment plan. This is true of medications, diets, and physical activity. Yes, there are general guidelines such as the 150-minutes-per-week rule based on several studies, but the important thing is that you should feel good after you exercise. Some people may be able to sleep extremely well after only a twenty-minute walk while others may need a full thirty minutes or even more to really notice a difference.

Most people will notice a significant boost in their mood after mild to moderate exercise, but for me, it is even more noticeable after a few bursts of high-intensity exercise, such as running a few fast intervals in the course of a longer moderate jog. This is when I really feel that runner's euphoria for hours afterward.

There is also no particular form of exercise that is perfect for every body, just as there is no one diet that works perfectly for everyone. I would encourage you to start with some kind of movement that you like, whether that is walking, biking, playing pickleball or soccer, taking dance classes, or starting tennis lessons. If your answer now is that there is no exercise that you enjoy, then it is time to go exploring. Try a couple weeks of classes at a gym, yoga studio, or martial arts dojo. Get outside or hop on a treadmill and take a walk. Join a pickup basketball game or soccer league. Keep exploring until you find the activity that makes you feel good and the time fly by.

If you are brand new or returning to exercise, those first few sessions will be the most difficult. It may take more than a day or two to find the joy in movement that I am describing, so there are some options to help with that as well. Of course you may be motivated by the idea that a better mood and a better night's sleep are just on the horizon (and hopefully you are by now). And you may be ready to tackle your first week knowing that after only a few sessions you'll be keyed into all the benefits mentioned. You can also help yourself get started by gamifying your activity, which is becoming an increasingly popular and more available means of motivation. Fitness trackers and watches offer encouragement in the form of badges, alerts, and rewards (and yet another jolt of dopamine to go with them). I particularly love closing my "fitness rings" every day. I also love that some video game platforms and virtual reality gaming devices now offer games that require movement to play. These games encourage exercise in place of an activity that has traditionally been completely sedentary, and as games do, they encourage the gamer to strive for one more goal, one more session, and they offer a tremendous sense of accomplishment in return.

Many sports also present an innate goal that may help motivate you to push through the initial hardship of getting started. It is amazingly easy to sweat for an extra few minutes when there is a point to be scored or a match to be won. We can almost forget that we are pushing our bodies to do something difficult when there is a reward coming soon! Adding a social aspect to exercise further augments the mental health benefits that we get from movement in addition to offering companions to keep us accountable and thus motivated to continue. This is also true of exercising with a class or a peer group. Sometimes after a long day, even if a workout session does not seem appealing initially, the chance to catch up with friends or teammates does, and it helps get us started until those feel-good chemicals kick in.

One of my patients who, like many busy working parents, found it difficult to squeeze in the time for exercise found that having it scheduled along with her children's activities helped to keep her consistent. She and a few other parents who would normally wait (and sit) while their kids participated in practices decided to start their own HIIT workout sessions nearby. They would be there at these scheduled times anyway and figured that they may as well get some exercise while their kids did. This made exercise a built-in part of the schedule as well as a group activity, so there were several reasons to show up.

Having your own goals and tracking them can also add some gamification to your routine, whether that comes in the form of hitting a milestone with your total miles logged for the month or the year, or a certain number of minutes or number of classes taken, or reaching a target such as completing a difficult set or mastering a particular yoga pose or dance movement. These short-term goals give us meaningful rewards, aside from the scale, that keep us motivated. Long-term goals should also be things other than weight, for instance accomplishing a certain number of repetitions or covering a distance in a certain amount of time. I have found that setting a goal of running a certain number of miles for the year keeps me going some mornings when I might otherwise be able to convince myself that it's too cold or that I'm too tired. These are goals that I have complete control over, even when the scale is bouncing around due to water-weight changes or a heavy meal. Goals and gamification can be powerful motivators.

Be a kid at heart! Remember that kids exercise all the time, and they think of it as *fun*, as play. What types of play did you enjoy when you were a child? Perhaps there is some long-forgotten joy ready to be tapped into. Maybe at some point you could no longer find the time for this activity, and it fell out of your usual routine. Or was there a reason that you got away from it? Maybe pain or injury stopped you from doing something that you loved when you were younger. If that's the case, and that pain or injury is still holding you back, then I recommend seeking medical attention. If you've recovered, maybe it's time to get back into it.

For those who may be even more reticent about starting a new workout regimen, the concept of "temptation bundling" may also be helpful. Professor Katherine Milkman from Wharton University studies this concept and coined the term.[42] Temptation bundling encourages new habits by pairing something we think we *should* do with something we really *want* to do. In her own personal example, Professor Milkman forced herself to exercise by riding a stationary bicycle while listening to audiobooks that she particularly looked forward to. In describing this personal journey, she stated that after a certain point she could not wait to get to the gym because her brain had become wired to expect a reward of juicy literature, so much so that she now found she looked forward to the gym as well. For my husband, this meant bundling treadmill time with a TV show that he had been wanting to watch. For some people, it's working out to a particular type of music or in some particular scenery, like paddleboarding in a beautiful lake at sunset. Whatever gets you looking forward to your exercise session, use it!

One of my patients swore to me that she would not enjoy any form

---

[42] Milkman, *How to Change*, 43.

of cardiovascular exercise we could possibly come up with. She, like many of my other patients, understood the importance of exercise, especially given her climbing cholesterol and blood pressure numbers, but she was adamant that she would never enjoy exercise. However, after a few more discussions, I learned that she did enjoy painting, and she had a lofted art studio in her backyard. We decided together that we could count painting as exercise if she stood while she did it and started painting on large canvases that required long arm movements. (This may have been an excuse to buy larger canvases, which I suspected she wanted to do anyway.) We also decided that she had to listen to fast-paced music while she painted to encourage large, fast movements, and that she had to do this for at least thirty minutes every day. It also helped that the studio was lofted above a garage, forcing her to climb a set of stairs every day. Three months after this discussion, she had lowered her blood pressure and cholesterol without adding any medication, and she actually lost some weight and inches off her waist and upper arms. But most importantly, she told me that she had so much more energy and was feeling great!

It's okay to start small. Studies investigating the mental health benefits of exercise have utilized a wide variety of exercise time and intensity in their study models, but positive outcomes are noted with even small amounts of exercise, like ten minutes a day, three days out of the week. As I mentioned earlier, most of the major studies aimed at reducing the risk of heart attack, stroke, diabetes, and elevated blood pressure use a model of 150 minutes of cardio exercise per week as the gold standard, and this is still the target that many clinicians advise. But if you, like many of my patients, hear that goal and feel that it is too daunting or too difficult to fit into your schedule, remember that five minutes is better than zero. Ten is even better than five, and so on. When you begin to feel the benefits that exercise offers to your sense of well-being, you will eventually start to crave more of it. It will come naturally. But it is okay to start off small at first, especially if that's what you have the time or stamina for at this moment.

Whatever motivates you to get started, use it! The boost of energy and better mood that you feel once you start should carry you the rest of the way to a lifelong healthy habit of activity.

But it is also important to be safe. If you are brand new to exercise, ease into it. If you are worried about a preexisting medical condition, talk to your medical provider before getting started. If you are worried about technique, you may want to work with a trainer or a coach. If you are worried about going it alone, find a friend to go with you. And remember to fuel and hydrate properly. The first few sessions of any new activity will be challenging, but remember that the entire point is ultimately to *feel good!*

Often the first five to ten minutes of exercise are the hardest. I have had many early-morning runs where, judging by my first mile, I thought that the day's workout might be cut short or that I might have to cut back my pace or intensity, but the body knows what we need and starts to deliver energy after those first few minutes of warming up. If I can manage to persist through that first mile or half mile, my legs start to feel lighter, my breathing gets easier, and running really does feel smoother.

My patients often ask about the best time of day to exercise. Several studies have looked at the benefits of exercise timing to evaluate whether there is an advantage to any particular time of day over another, and in general, there is very little data to suggest that the benefits are greater with any one time of day over others. However, in general, we do see that people who exercise at the beginning of their day tend to stay more consistent, and for that reason, many trainers and medical providers will recommend early-morning exercise.[43] Most importantly, get moving when it works for you and when you find that movement brings joy to your day.

---

[43] Schumacher et al., "Consistent Morning Exercise," 201–8.

CHAPTER 9

Food: Both Fuel and Pleasure

So far we have discussed only the effects of exercise or movement on our quality of life, and for good reasons that I hope are now obvious, but I would be remiss in discussing health if I left out the consideration of what we put into our bodies. There is a saying among fitness circles that "you can't outrun a bad diet." This is just as true for energy and mood as it is for weight. Food is necessary for fueling our activity and minds, and it can have a dramatic effect on how we feel in terms of mood, stamina, focus, sleep, and even physical pain. Food can bring its own pleasures too. A meal should leave you feeling good, good in your body and good about yourself.

Let's review a few quick key concepts regarding nutrition. Food provides energy and building materials for cells and for the chemicals that our bodies need to survive. Energy comes in the form of calories from carbohydrates, proteins, and fats. We also need proteins to provide the necessary ingredients for cell generation or repair. The food that we eat is either used for energy right away or stored for use later, thanks to the liver and the creation of adipose tissue (fat cells). When we go a long time without eating, for instance during an overnight fast, our liver reverses the storage process and breaks down the stored energy back into simple glucose to be used again. Our brains in particular are highly metabolically active and require lots of glucose, even during sleep, so we depend on this system of storage and release for survival.

So, the calories we consume provide us energy for now, and are also stored as energy for later. As mentioned at the beginning of this book, one pound of body fat equals roughly 3,500 excess calories, so if we eat that many extra calories over time, our body will build up one pound of fat storage, and if we burn off that many calories without replacing them, we will essentially lose one pound of body fat. These calories are composed of various macronutrients, measured in grams of proteins, carbohydrates, and fats. One gram of protein, for example, provides four calories of energy. One gram of carbohydrates also provides four calories of energy. However, fats provide nine calories per gram, which is one reason why low-fat diets became popular at several points throughout history. I remember the 1980s when sugary cereals were marketed as healthy since they were a low-fat food! The thinking was that reducing fat grams in the diet would lead to a reduction in calories overall. Most modern nutrition experts have rejected this way of thinking as many of these diets were not successful, and part of the reason for that is because fat grams also provide us with a sense of fullness. Carbohydrates, while imparting fewer calories per gram, do not trigger the same satiety response and make it easier for us to crave large portions before we feel satisfied.

I find that many of my patients who are focused solely on weight loss find it difficult to shed pounds through exercise alone. This is due in part to the fact that we tend to overestimate our total calorie burn and underestimate how much we consume. Remember that to lose one pound, we would have to run a deficit of 3,500 calories. For the average adult, exercise such as walking or running burns about one hundred calories per mile. So if you walk two miles, you would burn roughly two hundred calories. Of course, this will add up over time, so if you took that walk five times a week for an entire year, that would add up to fifty-two thousand calories! That's about fifteen pounds in a year. Now let's say you start to run instead of walk, and you cover three miles instead of two. Now you've burned three hundred calories per exercise session, and twenty-two pounds in a year. But all of that calorie burn can be negated pretty quickly with an extra postworkout snack or a high-calorie sports drink. So again, yes, we can lose pounds from exercise, but it takes time, and it may not happen at all if we increase our food intake after exertion.

Our bodies (and minds) tend to feel our best when we consume a variety of healthy foods and eat until we are sated but not necessarily stuffed. Eating past the point of satiety can cause significant pain and bloating, as most of us have probably experienced at one point or another in our lives, maybe during the holidays or at a festive event where the temptation to try all the delicious offerings is too great.

One might think that consuming a large amount of energy (calories) would leave us feeling, well . . . energetic! However, the digestive process diverts blood flow away from our muscles and other organs toward the gastrointestinal tract, so the majority of the energy we have available is used for the act of digestion. Our bodies also release a large amount of insulin, a hormone necessary for utilizing the glucose (sugars and other carbohydrates) we consume. However, especially in cases where we consume large portions, our bodies release so much insulin that the blood-sugar level, which initially spiked, will soon crash below our usual baseline. This leaves us feeling tired. (Think about that Thanksgiving afternoon nap time following a huge portion of potatoes, rolls, and pie.) And perhaps even more ironically, it also makes us crave sugars or carbohydrates all over again as our bodies work to get back to baseline.

In recent years, a new class of weight-loss medications have skyrocketed to fame precisely by lowering the threshold of this satiety response, even inducing nausea more readily in those who take the medication and then even slightly overindulge. These medications work by increasing the hormone normally made by our pancreas called GLP-1. In normal circumstances, our bodies release this chemical in response to food, and it functions to promote the release of other digestive enzymes, including insulin, amylase, and lipase, and by sending a signal to the brain that there is enough food present, and we're feeling full. So for people taking this medicine, it does become easier to consume smaller portions, which of course leads to weight loss, sometimes drastic weight loss. Our bodies still produce GLP-1 without this medication, and we can learn to tune in to our satiety signals more readily, which would not only help us slim down, but also to avoid those enormous portion sizes that make us lethargic.

When we focus solely on weight, we find a tendency to restrict nutrition, sometimes to an unhealthy extent. When I was at the peak of my swimming training, I felt that I had to constantly limit what I ate, a focus exacerbated by well-meaning coaches, one of whom advised restricting carbohydrates and calories to what I now know was a detrimental degree. After leaving swimming, I found myself increasingly fixated on those forbidden foods I "couldn't eat," so I would try to forswear them, but ultimately gave in to cravings and gained a large amount of weight. It took years to realize that by denying myself what I wanted to eat and choosing only what I thought was healthy, I was ultimately consuming large portions of things I didn't even want and left feeling unsatisfied. And then when I inevitably gave in to temptation, it felt like I had to shove down these forbidden foods so fast that I didn't even enjoy them, and I was left feeling horribly guilty afterward. At one point near the end of my undergraduate studies, I noticed that a close friend and classmate who seemed to effortlessly maintain a slim figure had very different habits than my own. If we went out to lunch, she would order whatever seemed appealing, but she often consumed only half of the portion that was served, or sometimes even less. And she always seemed satisfied at the end of the meal, whereas I sometimes left still thinking about the fried chicken I wish I had ordered instead of the lean salad. This is not to say that she ate completely unhealthy foods all the time. She definitely had fresh fruits and vegetables regularly. But if she wanted a burger or a slice of pizza, she would get it from time to time. She also listened to her body's satiety signals and stopped eating as soon as she was satisfied.

The other issue with extremely restrictive diet plans is that they do not work if they aren't sustainable. Some of my patients do experience initial success on a very restrictive diet, and they may lose ten, fifteen, or twenty pounds initially. But if the diet they have chosen is restrictive to the point that it doesn't fit into their lifestyle long term, then all of the initial weight loss quickly reverses.

I do have some patients who can give up bread, for instance, and live peacefully ever after. If that's the case for you, then go for it! But the majority of my patients, like me, would find that cooking for a family or having to eat while traveling makes it too difficult to restrict certain foods in the long term. We need a more sustainable approach.

We can take pleasure in our food while still recognizing how it makes our bodies feel. We can enjoy our coffee or tea while noticing that the timing of when we drink it is going to affect our sleep later. When we eat mindfully, we also tend to notice that greasy, fatty foods leave us feeling sluggish later; our guts become distended, and it becomes harder to breathe, harder to move, and harder to digest comfortably. So if you find yourself feeling this way, take notice of how you feel physically and remember that feeling for the next time you are faced with the decision of what or how much to eat. You may also notice that eating fresh fruits and vegetables or plain yogurt may leave you feeling better and still just as satisfied.

In the book *French Women Don't Get Fat*, author Mireille Guiliano discusses the pleasure of food.[44] She stresses that in taking the time to truly enjoy our meals, we ultimately do consume smaller portions. By contrast, food is often not associated with pleasure but with guilt, which is a most unhelpful emotion. We focus so much attention on what we think we should and should not eat and forget to be mindful of how our food makes us *feel*. When we focus on what our bodies truly need and want, we do make healthier decisions.

---

[44] Guiliano, *French Women Don't Get Fat*.

On the other hand, when we try to restrict our diets only to certain foods that we think we should eat, we often fall off of our plans (have a "cheat day" or a "cheat meal," as my patients would say), and we end up feeling guilty over it. Guilt is entirely unhelpful in this case. Scientists have shown that guilt creates the same stress-hormone release as other chronic stressors.[45] So for many of us who associate any pleasurable food with feelings of guilt or shame, those feelings cause a release of adrenaline and cortisol that actually interfere with digestion and seem to increase cravings for foods with high fat and sugar contents. We literally get stuck in a cycle of overindulging, feeling ashamed about it, and then eating more to manage the shame. It's no wonder that so many of my patients have a hard time breaking this cycle and finding a healthier diet that they feel good about and ultimately enjoy.

Food does offer its own sense of pleasure, and even a sense of reward. Of course, taste buds react pleasurably to delicious food, but the enjoyment does not stop there. When we consume something delicious, our brains release dopamine, the reward chemical we discussed earlier that gives us a sense of accomplishment, motivation, and even desire, sometimes to the point of addiction. Carbohydrates in particular seem to activate this dopamine release.[46] So when we talk about having a difficult time giving up sugar, it's no joke! Those carbohydrates are literally activating addiction signals in our brains, so eating a little something sweet can often make you feel even hungrier and want to consume more. This was likely helpful hundreds of years ago when periods of plenty were often followed by famine. Our bodies were able to take up all the excess fuel available and store it for later when seasons changed or harsh weather threatened the next year's food supply. But in most of the developed world in modern times, food scarcity is rarely an issue. Our bodies, however, have not adjusted to this new reality, so these

---

[45] Lupis et al., "Role of Shame and Body Esteem," 262–75.
[46] Thornley et al., "Carbohydrate Reward and Psychosis." 370–5.

cravings, the sense of addiction to sugar, carbohydrates, or salty, fatty foods, is a hard one to overcome.

This is precisely why lower carbohydrate diets work well for weight loss. It is not that carbohydrates are bad for us. In fact, fruits, vegetables, and whole grains have many important nutrients that our bodies need in order to be healthy. But the *amount* of food we eat when we consume carbohydrates, particularly processed, sugary carbohydrates, tends to increase greatly. As we ingest carbohydrates, our bodies quickly break them down into glucose to be used for energy. We experience a rapid rise in our blood-sugar levels. In response to this rise, our bodies release insulin, a hormone that allows the rest of the body's tissues, such as the muscles and liver, to utilize that glucose as energy. It essentially functions as the key that opens the doors (in this case the cell's channels) to let the sugar in. As the insulin rises, the glucose in the blood is used up and comes down. In the case of a high-carbohydrate or sugary meal, the rise in glucose occurs particularly quickly, and the insulin response is equally fast and robust to meet it, often overproducing just slightly so that the blood sugar comes down too quickly and drops to lower than ideal, causing us to experience a "sugar crash." In this state, we feel tired, moody, and even hungry! Our bodies send us signals that we need to bring the blood sugar (and dopamine level) back up again, and so we start to crave even more carbohydrates, and the cycle repeats. Breaking this cycle is extremely difficult, especially given how hardwired these cravings are.

By contrast, consuming fats tends to increase the release of hormones such as GLP-1 that signal satiety to our brains, one reason that high-fat, high-protein diets tend to promote weight loss. The fats are very filling, as opposed to carbohydrates, so we tend to consume fewer net calories. However, one of the pitfalls I find with high-fat diets is that many do not distinguish between types of fats. Processed foods with trans fats or foods high in saturated fats create a pro-inflammatory response in the body, which can trigger pain and discomfort as well as increased cholesterol and inflammatory factors. Healthy fats such as mono- and polyunsaturated fats, on the other hand, have the opposite effect. These are the types of fats found in nuts, seeds, olive oil, avocados, and fish like salmon or tuna. While every person's body responds differently to foods to some extent, I find that my body feels better when I eat more of these foods, and my patients report that they do too.

It is also important to incorporate protein into our meals, as these proteins contain the amino acids that the brain and body use to build peptides. These complex proteins are the building blocks for connective tissues like muscles and collagen but also chemicals like serotonin, dopamine, endorphins, and enkephalins. So consuming a variety of proteins is extremely important. However, there are serious flaws with these super-high-protein, low-carbohydrate diets as well. For one, our bodies do need some amount of carbohydrates for energy, and people on these diets often complain of feeling sluggish and tired from the lack of readily available energy in the form of glucose. Some of the literature encouraging these diets even tells people to avoid exercising, because it is a known fact that the body will not have enough energy to sustain even moderate physical activity. That fact alone should tell us that such a restrictive diet is not a good idea. Brain fog is another common complaint that I hear from my patients on these diets. This is because, like muscles, our brains are very metabolically active and require lots of energy in order to function well. Since the primary source of that energy comes directly from carbohydrates, our brains do need some carbohydrates to function optimally. In addition to the lack of fuel for our brains and muscles, some diets that are too high in protein can actually overtax the kidneys and lead to acute kidney injury, or in some cases, chronic kidney disease. Some high-protein sources are also high in saturated and trans fats, and again, diets with high fat content, particularly saturated fat, lead to a dramatic increase in LDL (or bad) cholesterol and eventually to a buildup of plaque in the arteries, increasing the risk for heart attack, blood clots, or strokes.

A poor diet can also be a major source of chronic inflammation. Some foods, especially foods high in sugars and trans fats, cause an increase in stress or inflammatory chemicals like cortisol.[47] Processed foods (like chips and candy) rank highly in this category. Processed meats like sausage and bacon also increase the inflammatory response. So if you eat mostly fast food or prepackaged or sugary snacks, your inflammatory response is chronically activated, ultimately making you feel not only bloated but also fatigued, and even anxious or depressed.

If you have ever given up certain inflammatory foods for a period of time (sugar, red meat, or alcohol for example) and then gone back and indulged, you've likely experienced the fatigue, the headaches, the overall malaise that comes from imbibing in these foods. If you have never tried going on an all-out sugar fast for a period of time, then I definitely recommend giving it some thought. The idea is not that you have to completely swear off sugar forever, for the rest of your life, but that you should at least have a sense of how these foods make you feel. A fast helps you get in touch with the effects that inflammatory food like sugar has on the body, on your energy level, on your sleep, and even on your physical pain.

On the other hand, some foods actually have anti-inflammatory effects on our bodies. Foods high in omega fatty acids like fish and walnuts rank highly in this category.[48] Fiber and carbohydrates that come from whole-grain sources (including fresh fruits and vegetables) rather than processed sugars and white flour also help to reduce the inflammatory response.

Anti-inflammatory diets have increased in popularity in recent years and are particularly popular among people who suffer from chronic-pain conditions such as arthritis or fibromyalgia. Some of my patients who suffer from these conditions but manage largely through lifestyle interventions can easily tell me when a holiday sugar crash or weekend of fast-food runs spurred their last flare-up.

---

[47] Ma et al., "Excessive Intake of Sugar," 988481.
[48] Dominguez et al., "Impact of Mediterranean Diet," 2028.

This is not to say that we can *never* have processed carbohydrates, sugars, or our other favorite treats. Part of feeling good is enjoying a treat every now and then, but we should be balancing these treats with how we feel when we eat them, and we realize fairly quickly that eating these things frequently does not help us to feel good. So yes, you can have a piece of cake at a birthday party or wedding celebration, but take your time and savor every bite of it. Enjoy it slowly, and you will probably find that you get plenty of enjoyment from a smaller portion or piece. You will also find that you know how much of these treats you can allow yourself to indulge in before feeling their negative physical effects. So you can have your splurge, and the following day, get back to your healthy routine without any sense of guilt or compulsion to compensate for yesterday's treats.

A diet that is rich in fresh produce, whole grains, healthy fats, and lean protein will give you the nutrients you need for better energy, mood, and sleep. And just as we focus on feeling good when we exercise, we should focus on how our food makes us feel as well. The taste and texture of food is pleasurable! Calming our hunger response is also pleasurable. At the end of a meal, we should be left with energy to move our bodies and exercise our minds in addition to feeling satisfied.

Balanced eating also means eating a variety of nutrients, including proteins, healthy fats, fruits, vegetables, and whole grains. These foods, especially when fresh and unprocessed, contain vitamins and minerals necessary for every bodily function. And eating healthy foods can be a source of pleasure too! This may take some practice and even some experimentation at first. If you, like so many of the patients I meet, rarely consume a vegetable in your day, you may experience some adjustment initially. Likewise, if you tend to consume an overabundance of sugar or saturated fats, you may not realize how sluggish these foods are making you feel until you learn to limit them. But even as you are limiting the foods that make you feel less than your best and learning to incorporate foods that satisfy your appetite and your body, you do not have to consider any particular food either all good or all bad. So it is not as if you can never enjoy a slice of pizza! In fact, if you truly want it, have a slice, and enjoy the heck out of it! And have a salad or some carrots and cucumber slices along with it. You should feel full and satisfied, but not bursting at the waistline. And if you overindulge on a particular occasion, it is not helpful to waste time chastising yourself. Rather, use it as an opportunity to make an observation: "I had too much [wine/sugar/grease/chips], and now I feel [bloated/hungover/sick/sleepy]. Next time I'll feel better if I have less of [this] or have [that] instead."

Just as there is no one particular form of exercise that works perfectly for every person, there is no one specific meal or diet that will work for everyone. Understandably, some people have diet restrictions based on allergy or intolerance to some foods, or even lifestyle choices due to moral or religious reasons. In general, we know that a healthy lifestyle includes limiting processed foods, which are high in preservatives, sugars, saturated fats, and sodium, and we need a variety of fresh and healthy nutrients. But within any of these parameters, it is possible to find a healthy, balanced diet that contributes to feeling *well*.

CONCLUSION

I feel that I cannot possibly overstate the benefits of a healthy lifestyle that have nothing to do with weight. A regular exercise routine will help you sleep better, feel happier, and enjoy better digestion and less pain, as well as decrease your blood pressure and blood sugar, lower your chance of developing heart disease, and reduce your risk of dementia or general cognitive decline. If these proven benefits were sold in the form of a pill or a shot, it would be impossible to keep in stock! But so many of us overlook these benefits and concentrate only on our weight or clothing size, and we give up when we don't see these improvements quickly enough.

I have often shared with patients that for me personally, exercise has to happen at five a.m. since I start work early. And at five o'clock in the morning, I could not possibly care less what the scale says or what size jeans I hope to be wearing that weekend. If these were my only goals, I would never get out of bed for that run. However, I *do* know even in my eyes-half-open state that if I get up and get at least a quick jog in before my day starts, I will be more focused and alert at work, in a brighter mood with my patients and coworkers, and more calm with my kids and spouse when I get home. Plus, I will sleep better the following evening. These immediate benefits will get me up and running in a way that no pair of skinny jeans ever will!

Along the way, my body has become more fit and more toned,

but much more important to me now than what my legs *look* like is what they can *do*. That sense of accomplishment, that sense of power, keeps me going as well.

I hope for each and every one of you that you find an activity that brings you joy and a sense of accomplishment, helps you handle daily stress, and makes you feel calmer, live happier, and sleep better. And yes, ultimately, you will be healthier by several metrics at your next check-up.

I am definitely not suggesting that anyone simply quit all of their medications and just pick up exercise and a mindful diet instead. But I will say to anyone and everyone that these practices will help you feel better and live a healthier life. Sure, you may be able to stop some medications eventually, but you should check with your medical provider before making any changes to your medical treatments. And remember, there are many medical conditions driven by genetics, and sometimes, even with efforts toward diet and exercise, the blood pressure will still be high, or the cholesterol will still not come down. These may be cases where we do need treatment, but needing medication is not a reason to give up on a healthy level of activity. There are so many more benefits to exercise that go beyond weight, cholesterol, or blood pressure.

Find an exercise or an activity that you enjoy and can do every day, and you will soon learn the excitement of seeing and feeling what your body can accomplish. When you truly feel good in your body, then ignore what the scale says! If, on the other hand, you know that you have not been getting much movement in your daily routine, and you are feeling listless, anxious, or tired frequently because of it, then it is time to get up and get moving. Focus on feeling good: having more energy, getting better sleep, and being in a better mood. The weight will likely come off with time, but even if it doesn't, the most important thing is that you will truly feel good and be healthier overall, with or without weight loss.

So many of my patients would say that "I felt great, but I just didn't see results, so I gave up." But we know, at a purely medical level, that there are so many benefits to exercise independent of weight loss, and even aside from the medical benefits, there are so many advantages that our patients can *feel* right away, and this can help us set habits for a healthier lifestyle. I have seen that change in so many of my patients, and it is just as motivating for me as it is for them.

My own husband—not a patient of mine, but whose health I bear in mind on a regular basis—was the one who finally convinced me to write all of this down and start getting the conversation out in the community. He had been an active runner earlier in life, but at one point fell prey to the busy working-parent lifestyle and neglected his regular exercise for quite some time. His primary care provider had encouraged him to increase physical activity, especially given his family history of high blood pressure and type 2 diabetes, but it never seemed to sink in. While jotting down some ideas for this book, I asked him to read a rough draft to get his thoughts on whether I should even proceed in writing more. He did not say much after reading it, but the next morning, he went on his first jog in several years. We all need to be reminded now and then how good we feel when our bodies are active, and that proved it!

I hope that all of you reading this (and my husband) find joy in your jogging sessions or whatever activity speaks to you, and that you continue a lifelong relationship with movement that makes you *feel good*.

ACKNOWLEDGMENTS

I could not have written this book without the amazing support of my husband, Joaquin, and my kids who encouraged me every day and also gave me the time and peace to write when I needed it.

I also have to thank my patients, who inspire me every day, especially those that allowed me to use their stories and examples in this book. I am truly blessed to work with and care for an incredible group of people!

And lastly, to my partners in exercise: my friend "CC," who inspired me to get back into running many years ago, as well as Missy, Will, and Stevie, who still join me for a jog or a walk around the trail now and then. Thank you for keeping the miles fun! To my favorite Pilates instructors, Donna and Emily, who have helped me find the strength and flexibility to stay injury-free in my other endeavors. And to my sailing community, who introduced me to my new favorite sport and have encouraged me through the muscle aches and "boat bites." Thank you for the tips and training and for introducing me to the best full-body workout in the most gorgeous settings!

BIBLIOGRAPHY

Allen, Jacob M., Lucy J. Mailing, Grace M. Niemiro, et al. "Exercise Alters Gut Microbiota Composition and Function in Lean and Obese Humans." *Medicine and Science in Sports and Exercise* 50, no. 4 (2018): 747–57. https://doi.org/10.1249/MSS.0000000000001495.

Alzheimer's Society. "Physical Activity and the Risk of Dementia." Accessed July 23, 2024. https://www.alzheimers.org.uk/about-dementia/managing-the-risk-of-dementia/reduce-your-risk-of-dementia/physical-activity.

Bailey, Tom G., N. Timothy Cable, Nabil Aziz, et al. "Exercise Training Reduces the Frequency of Menopausal Hot Flushes by Improving Thermoregulatory Control." *Menopause* 23, no. 7 (2016): 708–18. https://doi.org/10.1097/GME.0000000000000625.

Bastioli, Guendalina, Jennifer C. Arnold, Maria Mancini, et al. "Voluntary Exercise Boosts Striatal Dopamine Release: Evidence for the Necessary and Sufficient Role of BDNF." *Journal of Neuroscience* 42, no. 23 (2022): 4725–36. https://doi.org/10.1523/JNEUROSCI.2273-21.2022.

Biswas, A., P. I. Oh, G. E. Faulkner, et al. "Sedentary Time and Its Association with Risk for Disease Incidence, Mortality, and Hospitalization in Adults." *Annals of Internal Medicine* 162, no. 2 (January 2015): 123–32. https://doi.org/10.7326/M14-1651.

Brené, Stefan, Astrid Bjørnebekk, Elin Åberg, Aleksander A. Mathé, Lars Olson, and Martin Werme. "Running Is Rewarding and Antidepressive." *Physiology & Behavior* 92, no. 1–2 (2007): 136–40. https://doi.org/10.1016/j.physbeh.2007.05.015.

Couto, Nuno, Diogo Monteiro, Luís Cid, and Teresa Bento. "Effect of Different Types of Exercise in Adult Subjects with Fibromyalgia: A Systematic Review and Meta-Analysis of Randomized Clinical Trials." *Scientific Reports* 12 (2022): 10391. https://doi.org/10.1038/s41598-022-14213-x.

Dehnavi, Zahra Mohebbi, Farzaneh Jafarnejad, and Zahra Kamali. "The Effect of Aerobic Exercise on Primary Dysmenorrhea: A Clinical Trial Study." *Journal of Education and Health Promotion* 7, no. 1 (2018): 3. https://doi.org/10.4103/jehp.jehp_79_17.

Dominguez, Ligia J., Giovanna Di Bella, Nicola Veronese, and Mario Barbagallo. "Impact of Mediterranean Diet on Chronic Non-Communicable Diseases and Longevity." *Nutrients* 13, no. 6 (2021): 2028. https://doi.org/10.3390/nu13062028.

Eaton, Katherine, Floyd R. Sallee, and Renu Sah. "Relevance of Neuropeptide Y (NPY) in Psychiatry." *Current Topics in Medicinal Chemistry* 7, no. 17 (2007): 1645–59. https://doi.org/10.2174/156802607782341037.

Ebner, Karl, Nadia M. Rupniak, Alois Saria, and Nicolas Singewald. "Substance P in the Medial Amygdala: Emotional Stress-Sensitive Release and Modulation of Anxiety-Related Behavior in Rats." *Proceedings of the National Academy of Sciences of the United States of America* 101, no. 12 (2004): 4280–5. https://doi.org/10.1073/pnas.0400794101.

Elwood, Peter, Julieta Galante, Janet Pickering, et al. "Healthy Lifestyles Reduce the Incidence of Chronic Diseases and Dementia: Evidence from the Caerphilly Cohort Study." *PLOS One* 8, no. 12 (2013): https://doi.org/10.1371/journal.pone.0081877.

Ennour-Idrissi, Kaoutar, Elizabeth Maunsell, and Caroline Diorio. "Effect of Physical Activity on Sex Hormones in Women: A Systematic Review and Meta-Analysis of Randomized Controlled

Trials." *Breast Cancer Research* 17 (November 2015): 139. https://doi.org/10.1186/s13058-015-0647-3.

Erickson, Kirk I., Michelle W. Voss, Ruchika Shaurya Prakash, et al. "Exercise Training Increases Size of Hippocampus and Improves Memory." *Proceedings of the National Academy of Sciences of the United States of America* 108, no. 7 (2011): 3017–22. https://doi:10.1073/pnas.1015950108.

Fani, Mozhgan, Javid Mostamand, Maedeh Fani, Navid Chitsaz, and Awat Feizi. "The Effect of Aerobic Exercises Among Women with Mild and Moderate Irritable Bowel Syndrome: A Pilot Study." *Journal of Bodywork and Movement Therapies* 23, no. 1 (2019): 161–5. https://doi:10.1016/j.jbmt.2018.02.003.

Francis, K. "The Role of Endorphins in Exercise: A Review of Current Knowledge." *The Journal of Orthopaedic and Sports Physical Therapy* 4, no. 3 (1983): 169–73. https://doi.org/10.2519/jospt.1983.4.3.169.

Fransen, Marlene, Sara McConnell, Alison R. Harmer, Martin Van der Esch, Milena Simic, Kim L Bennell. "Exercise for Osteoarthritis of the Knee: A Cochrane Systematic Review." *British Journal of Sports Medicine* 49, no. 24 (2015):1554–7. https://doi.org/10.1136/bjsports-2015-095424.

Guiliano, Mireille. *French Women Don't Get Fat.* Vintage, 2006.

Hanna, Fahad, Emily You, and Mohamed El-Sherif. "Editorial: The Impact of Sedentary Behavior and Virtual Lifestyle on Physical and Mental Wellbeing: Social Distancing from Healthy Living." *Frontiers in Public Health* 11 (2023): 1265814. https://doi.org/10.3389/fpubh.2023.1265814.

Harshitha, Shanmugam, Emilio Molina Molina, Domenica Maria Di Palo, et al. "Physical Activity Modulating Lipid Metabolism in Gallbladder Diseases." *Journal of Gastrointestinal and Liver Diseases* 29, no. 1 (2020): 99–110. https://doi.org/10.15403/jgld-544.

Iso-Markku, Paula, Urho M. Kujala, Keegan Knittle, Juho Polet, Eero Vuoksimaa, Katja Waller. "Physical Activity as a Protective Factor for Dementia and Alzheimer's Disease: Systematic Review, Meta-Analysis and Quality Assessment of Cohort and Case-Control Studies." *British Journal of Sports Medicine* 56, no. 12 (2022): 701–9. https://doi:10.1136/bjsports-2021-104981.

Johannesson, Elisabet, Gisela Ringström, Hasse Abrahamsson, and Riadh Sadik. "Intervention to Increase Physical Activity in Irritable Bowel Syndrome Shows Long-Term Positive Effects." *World Journal of Gastroenterology* 21, no. 2 (2015): 600–8. https://doi.org/10.3748/wjg.v21.i2.600.

Karrer, Teresa M. "Reduced Dopamine Receptors and Transporters but Not Synthesis Capacity in Normal Aging Adults: A Meta-Analysis." *Neurobiology of Aging* 57 (September 2017): 36–46. https://doi.org/10.1016/j.neurobiolaging.2017.05.006.

Kienast, Camilla, Hanns-Christian Gunga, and Mathias Steinach. "Neuropeptide Y – Its role in Human Performance and Extreme Environments." *Reach* 14, nos. 14–15 (2019): 10032. https://doi.org/10.1016/j.reach.2019.100032.

Kivipelto, Miia, Alina Solomon, Satu Ahtiluoto, et al. "The Finnish Geriatric Intervention Study to Prevent Cognitive Impairment and Disability (FINGER): Study Design and Progress." *Alzheimer's & Dementia: The Journal of the Alzheimer's Association* 9, no. 6 (2013): 657–65. https://doi:10.1016/j.jalz.2012.09.012.

Lima, Lucas V., Thiago S. S. Abner, Kathleen A. Sluka. "Does Exercise Increase or Decrease Pain? Central Mechanisms Underlying These Two Phenomena." *The Journal of Physiology* 595, no. 13 (2017): 4141–50. https://doi.org/10.1113/JP273355.

Lupis, Sarah B., Natalie J. Sabik, and Jutta M. Wolf. "Role of Shame and Body Esteem in Cortisol Stress Responses." *Journal of Behavioral Medicine*, 39 no. 2 (2015): 262–75. https://doi.org/10.1007/s10865-015-9695-5.

Ma, Xiao, Fang Nan, Hantian Liang, et al. "Excessive Intake of Sugar: An Accomplice of Inflammation." *Frontiers in Immunology* 13 (August 2022): 988481. https://doi.org/10.3389/fimmu.2022.988481.

Mailing, Lucy J., Jacob M. Allen, Thomas W. Buford, Christopher J. Fields, Jeffrey A. Woods. "Exercise and the Gut Microbiome: A Review of the Evidence, Potential Mechanisms, and Implications for Human Health." *Exercise and Sport Sciences Reviews* 47, no. 2 (2019): 75–85. https://doi.org/10.1249/JES.0000000000000183.

Malesu, Vijay Kumar. "The Link Between Cortisol, Inflammation, and Disease." *Medical Life Sciences News*, accessed March 30, 2025. https://www.news-medical.net/health/The-Link-Between-Cortisol-Inflammation-and-Disease.aspx.

Marchant, David, Sophie Hampson, Lucy Finnigan, Kelly Marrin, Craig Thorley. "The Effects of Acute Moderate and High Intensity Exercise on Memory." *Frontiers in Psychology* 11, (July 2020): 1716. http://doi:10.3389/fpsyg.2020.01716.

Pagliusi, Marco Jr., and Felipe V. Gomes. "The Role of the Rostral Ventromedial Medulla in Stress Responses." *Brain Sciences* 13, no. 5 (2023): 776. https://doi.org/10.3390/brainsci13050776.

Marusak, Hilary A. "The 'Runner's High' May Result from Molecules Called Cannabinoids – The Body's Own Version of THC and CBD." *Today@Wayne*, Wayne State University, January 3, 2022. https://today.wayne.edu/news/2022/01/03/the-runners-high-may-result-from-molecules-called-cannabinoids-the-bodys-own-version-of-thc-and-cbd-46709.

Mawe, Gary M., and Jill M. Hoffman. "Serotonin Signalling in the Gut—Functions, Dysfunctions and Therapeutic Targets." *Nature Reviews Gastroenterology & Hepatology* 10, no. 8 (2013): 473–86. https://doi.org/10.1038/nrgastro.2013.105

Milkman, Katherine. *How to Change: The Science of Getting from Where You Are to Where You Want to Be.* Penguin Publishing Group, 2021.

Mischel, Walter. *The Marshmallow Test: Mastering Self-Control.* Brilliance Audio, 2014.

Morita, Emiko, Hisayo Yokoyama, Daiki Imai, et al. "Aerobic Exercise Training with Brisk Walking Increases Intestinal Bacteroides in Healthy Elderly Women." *Nutrients* 11, no. 4 (2019): 868. https://doi.org/10.3390/nu11040868.

Mudge, A. W., Leeman, S. E., and Fischbach, G. D. "Enkephalin Inhibits Release of Substance P from Sensory Neurons in Culture and Decreases Action Potential Duration." *Proceedings of the National Academy of Sciences of the United States of America* 76, no. 1 (1979): 526–30. https://doi.org/10.1073/pnas.76.1.526.

National Cancer Institute: Surveillance Epidemiology and End Results (SEER) Program. "Annual Report to the Nation 2022 National Cancer Statistics." Accessed October 2, 2024. https://seer.cancer.gov/report_to_nation/statistics.html.

Nys, Len De, Kerry Anderson, Esther F. Ofosu, Gemma C. Ryde, Jenni Connelly, and Anna C. Whitaker. "The Effects of Physical Activity on Cortisol and Sleep: A Systematic Review and Meta-Analysis." *Psychoneuroendocrinology* 143 (September 2022): 105843. https://doi.org/10.1016/j.psyneuen.2022.105843.

Rudolph, D. L., and E. McAuley. "Cortisol and Affective Responses to Exercise." *Journal of Sports Sciences* 16, no. 2 (1998): 122–8. https://doi.org/10.1080/026404198366830.

Schumacher, Leah M., J. Graham Thomas, Hollie A. Raynor, Ryan E. Rhodes, Dale S. Bond. "Consistent Morning Exercise May Be Beneficial for Individuals with Obesity." *Exercise and Sport Sciences Reviews* 48, no. 4 (2020), 201–8. https://doi.org/10.1249/JES.0000000000000226.

Shele, Grei, Jessica Genkil, and Diana Speelman. "A Systematic Review of the Effects of Exercise on Hormones in Women with Polycystic Ovary Syndrome." *Journal of Functional Morphology and Kinesiology* 5, no. 2 (2020): 35. https://doi.org/10.3390/jfmk5020035.

Thaler, Richard H. *Misbehaving*. W. W. Norton, 2016.

Thornley, Simon, Bruce Russell, and Rob Kydd. "Carbohydrate Reward and Psychosis: An Explanation for Neuroleptic Induced Weight Gain and Path to Improved Mental Health?" *Current Neuropharmacology* 9, no. 2 (2011): 370–5. https://doi.org/10.2174/157015911795596513.

Trevino, Colleen M., Timothy Geier, Rachel Morris, Susan Cronn, and Terri deRoon-Cassini. "Relationship Between Decreased Cortisol and Development of Chronic Pain in Traumatically Injured." *Journal of Surgical Research* 270 (February 2022): 286–92. https://doi.org/10.1016/j.jss.2021.08.040.

Vahora, Ilmaben S., Nicholas Tsouklidis, Rajat Kumar, Ravi Soni, and Safeera Khan. "How Serotonin Level Fluctuation Affects the Effectiveness of Treatment in Irritable Bowel Syndrome." *Cureus* 12, no. 8 (2020): e9871. https://doi.org/10.7759/cureus.c36.

Weeldreyer, Nathan R., Jeison C. De Guzman, Craig Paterson, Jason D. Allen, Glenn A. Gaesser, Siddhartha S. Angadi. "Cardiorespiratory Fitness, Body Mass Index and Mortality: A Systematic Review and Meta-Analysis." *British Journal of Sports Medicine* 59 (February 2025): 339–46. https://doi.org/10.1136/bjsports-2024-108748.

Young, Simon N. "How to Increase Serotonin in the Human Brain Without Drugs." *Journal of Psychiatry and Neuroscience* 32, no. 6 (2007): 394–9. https://pmc.ncbi.nlm.nih.gov/articles/PMC2077351.

Zong, Boyi, Fengzhi Yu, Xiaoyou Zhang, et al. "Understanding How Physical Exercise Improves Alzheimer's Disease: Cholinergic and Monoaminergic Systems." *Frontiers in Aging Neuroscience* 14 (May 2022): 869507. https://doi.org/10.3389/fnagi.2022.869507.

www.ingramcontent.com/pod-product-compliance
Lightning Source LLC
LaVergne TN
LVHW092054060526
838201LV00047B/1386